DEPRA

Renata Ažman

DEPRA

Celjska Mohorjeva in conjunction with DAM, The
Society for Individuals Suffering from Depression
and Anxiety Disorders

Renata Ažman

All rights reserved, no part of this publication may be reproduced by any means, electronic, mechanical, or photocopying, documentary, film, or otherwise without prior permission of the publisher.

>Published by:
>Chipmunkapublishing
>PO Box 6872
>Brentwood
>Essex
>CM13 1ZT
>United Kingdom

http://www.chipmunkapublishing.com

Copyright © 2007 Renata Ažman

Cover Image: Marie Berger
Edited: Jože Faganel

DEPRA

Foreword

I met Renata Azman two years ago on the Slovenian Coast at Portoroz. Introduced by a mutual friend we quickly discovered a common interest in the lived experiences of people who had acquired a psychiatric diagnosis. The vivid and engaging way in which Renata talked to me about what she was writing about her own experiences left me eager to read her work. At the end of our time together I encouraged her to consider sharing some of her experiences and expertise with an English speaking audience. This was not just to satisfy my need to learn more, I thought that others could learn a lot from sharing her journey through the ups and downs of emotional distress.

Two years later Renata has taken this step, through this edition of Depra, a book that has attracted considerable interest and acclaim in Slovenia. In the country of Renata's birth Depra has succeeded in opening up a world of experience that has been absent largely absent from the academic literature of mental health. For far too long it has been mental health professionals-psychiatrists, psychologists and nurses who have dominated the field of published articles and books about mental health. Their work has been based on their observations and interpretations of those that they have diagnosed as mentally ill.

Renata Ažman

Depra redresses the balance by adding to the growing body of literature from 'the other side'. The literature of people who have found themselves subject to the scrutiny and interventions of mental health professionals. Mental health service users and survivors of the psychiatric system who are opening up their experiences to others free from the commentaries of those who claim to 'know what is best' for them . Reading Depra will take you to a place where you can learn directly about what it means to struggle, survive and find ways of moving forwards and take your place in the world.

In Europe, at the moment, it is estimated that 1 in 4 citizens will experience emotional distress at some time in their lives, severe enough to result in a psychiatric diagnosis. Alongside the problems of dealing with the impact of living with changing emotional states, these individuals will find themselves facing the prejudice, discrimination and the abuse of their human rights which are associated with society's responses to 'the mentally ill' . Whilst it is important to understand and respect the ethnic, spiritual, gender, sexuality, class and age diversities that shape us as individuals it is also important to recognise some of the commonalities of experience that shape our lives and who we are. It is from books like this one that we are reminded that experiences of emotional distress are not those of 'the other' but are ones to which we can all make a connection and in doing so need to recognise our

DEPRA

common humanity. It is from books like this that we can learn about how individual service users as well as service user organisations can contribute to our understandings of the responses that can be made to address mental health problems.

As the Director of a University based Centre of Excellence in Interdisciplinary Mental Health that is founded on the principal that the knowledge of those using mental health services is of equal value to the knowledge base of those working in and researching mental health, I commend this book as one which makes an important contribution to the knowledge we need if we are to build a responsive, socially just and humane response to mental distress in the twenty first century.

Professor Ann Davis
Director CEIMH (www.ceimh.bham.ac.uk)
Birmingham August 2007

Renata Ažman

DEPRA

Contents

J. Magdič: Foreword
R. Ažman: Depra
      I. Who am I? Where am I going?
      II. Diary.
      III. Healer.
      IV. Thanks, God.
A. Marušič: Depression is just an illness

Renata Ažman

DEPRA

Foreword

Dear readers!

I've been a psychiatrist for 35 great years, and thank God for them. I mention this, because in all this time, I have never come across such an open psychology book as this one by Renata Ažman. I've read many psychiatry books, but on the other hand I owe a great deal to my "patients'" understanding of their psyche. Many people suffering mental problems teach psychiatrists more than many a textbook. Renata Ažman's book is a combination of a psychiatry book and her personality. It discusses her psyche scientifically. Should any theologians be reading my words, I can tell them that I've deliberately used the words psyche and soul; I am not mixing these two terms. As a medical psychiatrist, I'd rather stick to psyche, but the depth of Renata's writing extends to the realm of the soul, and not just hers, but my own.

I am proud that I can help with Renata Ažman's book. To me she is not a patient in any disparaging sense of the word, since I am not someone "better", some therapist standing over her. We are all patients, martyrs to this life, which has only two sides: either you

Renata Ažman

need help, or you give it. You decide. But in our lives, these two roles switch.

Look into yourself, dear reader, not into someone else, not into the psyche of Renata Ažman, but I repeat, into yourself. Renata tells me this too, since otherwise I couldn't read her expertly described mental state. This excellent book is a description of the "psychic status" of us psychiatrists – that is her work. This book forces readers into longitudinal, in-depth reflection on themselves. You recognise that there were times in your life when you turned upwards, and then there are times when you shed an ocean of tears. I hope that for you, dear reader, everything worked out well. I hope it will, if it hasn't already. Renata describes her mental state in depth, talks about "her" incurable illness. Mania will follow depression, and so it will be until the end. Renata sees, experiences her mental breadth. Her ego experiences swings between the banks of her feelings.

"Depression is a devil," says Renata. I know, Renata, that this is also true of mania, which is not heaven, but also a devil. Renata's heart is used to tears, "There've been so many, with more to come, but it doesn't matter". Such understanding and dedication brings tears to my eyes. Renata gratefully points out the status of being satisfied with an "average" situation, how happy she would be "in an ordinary person's shoes". She wants a few years without depression and without fear.

DEPRA

What do psychiatrists actually do? How and to what extent do we understand, treat, cure depression? Renata shows us. She comes to be in the same state, on the same level, as a psychiatrist. You just have to listen. Visitors to my practice often themselves provide the guidelines for my "professional action".

It's true, dear Renata, animals are not as self-destructive as people. So-called individuation doesn't always make you happy. The tree of knowledge expelled Adam and Eve from Eden. Knowledge, understanding of oneself places a person in the position of God, but what if there's no God?. Standing on a cliff is not good, not sustainable, it's a form of narcissism. It's good to dive into the waters of your own mental interior. Here too is the meaning of depression in its therapeutic sense. What am I saying? When I was studying at the Jung Institute in Zurich, the head of the institute said: "God, give you depression". What would Renata say to that? There is no understanding without going deep into yourself, dear Renata. But what Renata has in excess, namely depression, many people could use in their questionable real actions.

The just Renata, like the biblical Job, is debating with God. She does not condemn God, she does not curse him. She experiences God in his breadth, as her psyche is broad. "God recognises all truths, including the truth that there is no God." Job's story in our understanding has a happy ending. God, let Renata be happy too. On

Renata Ažman

this journey, she found in herself "a frail child". What a profound psychological truth. Jung's psychology talks of the inner child, as a therapeutic factor on our "tramp's journey". People, I beg you, don't destroy the child within! For senex there is still time, even if we're already in the second half of life. What is the time of a human life in the light of Chronos, is there even a boundary between puer and senex? In depression, Renata's ego fights for "every centimetre of my brain". How well she knows the role of the brain in depressive incidents. She offers the reader a self-help approach, how to hold the ego above the water. She finds that, in depression, a person is incapable of rational consideration of the "logical". Depression is an "illness" of the emotions, with "negative feelings" dominating the ego. If reason was still able to drag the cart out of the swamp, there would be no depression. But every pit has its floor. Renata is emerging from depression, is recognising and thinking, so she has a chance to come to an idea, thinking, mental functioning that brings us closest to reality. Towards the end of the book, Renata – rationally and deserving of praise – becomes a psychotherapist. She gives real instructions for the journey from night to day. She does not condemn the world for her state. "The world is good and bad, black and white, and a whole range of shades in between." To these, Renata's words, I add my own: the world is manic and depressive, and in between there is a whole palette of shades. The peak of her psychotherapeutic gift is placing parents at the heart,

DEPRA

"Love your children." Love is the basis of the joy of life.

Dear Renata! My heartfelt thanks for this book!

Dr. Jožef Magdič, specialist psychiatrist

Renata Ažman

DEPRA

I.

Who am I? Where am I going?

God's blessing on all nations,
Who long and work for that bright day,
When o'er earth's habitations
No war, no strife shall hold its sway;
Who long to see
That all men free
No more shall foes, but neighbours be.

So France[1] wrote. I read somewhere recently that he drank a lot. God knows why. Maybe if I knew more of his story, I could understand him better. There's a lot been written about him, but how much of it is true, only he knew. Everybody knows best their own story, their own cross and their own fate. *And each of us is only one of us.*

I talked to my psychiatrist yesterday. She told me that I've not just got manic-depressive psychosis, but also schizo-affective disorder. Fine. That too. No problem. Right now I'm battling depression. Want to know how I'm doing?

---

[1] France Prešeren, Slovenia's national poet.

Renata Ažman

Connections.

Connections. You think they're there, and then you see they're not. One minute they're back, next minute they're gone again. If you're on your own with nothing to tie you down, you can cope with it. Oliver left today. My dog. He's in good hands. I can't afford a vet. I cry whenever I think of him. Oliver loved me, but sadly he was always ill. And hungry. I couldn't cope. I cry. This book will mostly talk about depression, a place I'm slowly but surely heading towards. When you're depressed, your brain doesn't function properly, so this book is not a melodic novel of life, but a bunch of thoughts that – in this difficult and painful time – I managed to gather together and condense into a few sentences. I do hope, though, that through them I can take you at least to the entrance to the gloomy cavern called depression. Depression – at least for me – is followed by mania and so on. My illness is incurable. This is how it's going to be until the end. Maybe a happy end, who knows? When I die, I want to be alone with God. *And the angels*. And I want it to be at night. Then I can die. One day I will. I don't know. I'm more afraid of life.

Every day the fear is worse. God help me.
Easter Sunday. Ham and eggs, *potica*[2] and the like for breakfast. The roads are busy. Slovenes are travelling, enjoying themselves. Lucky for them; they've got

---

[2] A traditional Slovenian cake.

DEPRA

somewhere to go. I'll be fine at home. I have to clean the flat. Tomorrow's another holiday. I'll bet the shopping centres are packed again today. But if they're shut, this is going to be another black weekend. If people are off work and at home together for too long, it's not long before the arguments start. No, holidays are not for everyone. At peace and in the spirit of the holiday, I finally got round to watching Mel Gibson's The Passion of the Christ. Horrible. Really horrible. And if you ask me, a little too realistic. Crucifixion is a horribly painful way to die. And Jesus was flogged, and made to wear the crown of thorns. They mocked him, and tortured him brutally. Cruelly. It's Thursday today, and tomorrow is the first of April.
Pope John Paul the Second died today. Honour his memory, he was a great man.

God help me.
I'm not well, I'm tired.
God help me. Depression's pumping through my veins.
Please don't let it last too long. Pleeeaase.

I worked as a proper reporter today for the first time in ages. The Belarussian winner of the Eurovision song contest came to Slovenia today with her tycoon husband. I wrote, filed the report, thirty *juri*[3], loaded. Now I can go to the shops. I was wondering the other day why we've fallen so deep into consumerist post-capitalism, and I realised that it often feels like

---

[3] *Juri*, Slovenian slang for a thousand tolars.

everything's going on behind our backs. Like a horoscope. This week's the same for all Aquarians? Come on!.

Ratzinger's the new pope. A German. God, let him rule wisely. Benedict the Sixteenth. Cool.

Misery, black and uninvited.

A lot of very sad things have happened in my life. I don't want to think about them, but sometimes dark thoughts swamp my brain. Misery. When it comes round the corner, black and uninvited, it's terrible. I've got so many reasons to be sad. It'll pass. My heart has grown used to tears. There've been so many, with more to come, but it doesn't matter.

I know who I am, but I don't know where I'm going and how all of this will end. But like I said, there's no way back. Sometimes it really did used to be better, with no telephones or any of this Internet shit. You sit in front of the computer, times passes, you lie to yourself that you're doing something useful, and the days, weeks, months all pass. And not just that. What about your back? Your eyes? And your general well-being? We used to go for walks, now we chat online. Is this normal?

Andrej once told me that once you've set out on the path of transformation, there's no way back. So it's

DEPRA

pointless to look back on old patterns and ways of thinking; it's better to spend your energy on new knowledge. For some time now I've had the feeling that depression teaches me that I can sometimes see the world differently. I believe that each of us has an inbuilt code to understand the world. And if you find it, you've made it. All too often though, we simply adopt the code of our parents and relatives, forgetting about our own. And this is the key to understanding the world and the universe around us. Everyone must find their own path, whatever it may be.

... Remember me when I am gone away,
Gone far away into the silent land;
When you can no more hold me by the hand.

War.
I'm watching an old video – a Djordje Balašević[4] concert in the Sava Centre in Belgrade on 6 January 1994, and I'm listening in amazement and respect to all the sketches and jokes which at the time – during the war – sounded very different from now. Or before, before all of this. The madness of war, ethnic cleansing, mass murder and extreme nationalism were things we only got used to during the war. We were taught differently at school, so we didn't really know what the word war meant. It's completely different if you experience it first hand. Then you understand, but not before.

---

[4] A well-known Serbian singer-songwriter.

Renata Ažman

Yes, it was a dirty war. All the worst aspects of human nature erupted onto the scene. I read somewhere that there is a killer in each of us; a torturer and a torture victim, a saint and a hangman. Many innocent people died horribly in this Balkan war. All the Balkan wars have been bloody, but it's not just Balkan wars – all wars are bloody. They're very successful, they inflame spirits and martial passions incited by politicians and war profiteers. The saddest thing is, in the end there's no winner. Nobody has anything to celebrate.
Yesterday I wrote a little poem. Sometimes it helps me get through the day. Sometimes.

Illusion?

If everything my heart feels,
my eyes see,
is but an illusion,
then I too
am but an illusion
in the middle of the night.

I know it's amateurish, but every beginning is difficult.
This time it's for real.
I spoke to Niveska today. Niveska lives in Cologne near the cathedral, but she spends her summers in her house in the little Dalmatian village of Murvica on Brač. I've spent a lot of time there, so we've become

close and know each other well; now we call each other from time to time, and chat about how we're feeling; sometimes we laugh a lot. Niveska is seventy-nine, but she's still in great form. She doesn't think about her age, she lives like she's thirty. And she definitely never moans. At least less she moans than I do. She always finds a comforting word when I need one. She also knows what depression is. She experienced it herself, and I have the feeling that she respects me more since then. All of her friends are slightly crazy, and I'm proud that she counts me as one of them.

Age is just an illusion. That's why they say you're only as old as you feel. I know lots of very lively old people who don't complain, but enjoy themselves as far as their health will allow. I'd like to be as old as some of them.

In the name of love.

Today Pope Benedict the Sixteenth will address the faithful for the first time from the balcony on St Peter's Square. I'd really like to know whether the doves, the birds of peace, will listen to him too. If the Pope is God's emissary on Earth, then he's certainly equally close to all the living creatures that God created. Even doves. I see them every day, and I don't like them. Often, the doves I watch through the window are the only living creatures I see all day. When I'm depressed, I don't go out, so the view of the concrete beam on which the doves sit is my only window on the world.

Renata Ažman

There's lots of doves in cities, especially in Italy. I went to Florence and Assisi once. Having paid my two euros, I was standing looking at Leonardo's painting – I could even touch it – when I realised that I too am now part of this majestic world of art, never fully knowable. There's always something left unsaid, there's always an unanswered question at the end. And that's the magic of it. You're always investigating and learning, and that's beautiful. That's how I got to know Leonardo da Vinci for one. Francis of Assisi for another. We got to Assisi – I was with a couple of friends – about six in the evening. We had a look around and then slept well in a nearby car park. I woke up about five in the morning, and ended up waiting for sunrise in a small car park below the crag on which stands the Church of St Francis of Assisi. I was always a fan of St Francis. When I entered the room where his relics are kept, I had a strange realisation. For the first time I realised that angels never die. Ever since then, Assisi to me has been the most beautiful place in the world. Whenever I'm in a bad way, I grab the album and look at the photos. Sometimes, when things are bad, the energy of such a beautiful memory takes the pain away for a minute or two. And that's like an oasis in the middle of the desert: sometimes it's worth more than all the treasure in the world.

DEPRA

God, help me. Help.

You were born for me,
You are fated for me,
For me to love you in my heart,
For me to carry you in my eye ...

Today's a difficult day. Depression is pumping through my veins, every day is darker than the last. I pray it won't last long this time. I need a shower; maybe then I'll feel a bit better. Water's always good for the body, inside and out. It takes away all the negative energy that builds up in our energy centres throughout the day. Life is energy, which flows from one to another, and then on to a third ... the mere interaction of energy, nothing more. No more, no less. The most beautiful energy is the energy of love. Only love can heal mental anguish, including depression. There's as much love in the world as there is in our hearts. That's the key to understanding the world, and I now know what the Little Prince meant when he said that you have to look with your heart. You have to feel everything around you. Space, objects, plans, animals, people, God. Everything in the world has its energy, and if Einstein is right, energy is indestructible. Such then is our mortal life.

Renata Ažman

... how can I put it? The energy of the sky and the horizon will meld into one and then in your heart you will feel the love ... of this world and the other.

I feel it every day: the love of this world and the other. I feel it heal me; I sense how it will heal me. Love is one and indivisible. And it must be respected and cared for, just like you care for a little baby that's not yet got its first tooth. Many bad things have happened in the name of love, but that wasn't real love. It didn't know how to, it wouldn't, it couldn't be real love. Such love, real and unconditional, is God's love. Some people are also capable of such love, but of course most aren't. And I always wanted to be one of the former. Always.

DEPRA

II.
Diary.

I was very scared again yesterday. Once again I felt in my bones the despair that hits me whenever I'm depressed. The fear grows minute by minute; every step is a step in the dark. A horrible feeling. But it seems eventually I'll have to come to terms with the fact that there will always be fear in my life. When it's really bad, I take a Xanax, and things are a little better. Am I doing the right thing?

Act only according to that maxim whereby you can at the same time will that it should become a universal law.

Kant's categorical imperative. Politicians in particular should apply it, and strive for a more just world. At least while they're in office. Politics is always superior in its relations to other areas of human life. Whenever anything falls apart, politicians always have the last word; unfortunately, they don't realise it. They don't realise their responsibility, or that their function is honourable and they should perform it honourably. But they only look out for themselves – and for sure, not just Slovenian politicians – to make money and contacts that will help them in later life and increase their power. The world would be a much better place if people lived more modestly, honestly and with good intentions. Things could be beautiful in our unhappy world. But they're not. Everybody looks out for themselves, and sometimes the feeling you can't change anything, and that you can't trust anybody, is unbearable. Maybe that's just my paranoia though. I don't know.

Do you remember how ...

Life on Earth is in fact a great phenomenon. If there is someone – some higher intelligence – watching over us up in the sky, they certainly have an opinion about us. Maybe there is someone secretly marvelling at us, but they're just as likely to be laughing at us. People really are funny. We embitter life, ourselves, and each other. Why?
But things could be so beautiful.
Today I actually feel tolerable. But that doesn't mean anything. By tomorrow I might be obscured by dark clouds, having to fight for every breath, every word, every sentence that I want to put on paper. I hope the angels are with me then.

Diego died. I can't believe it. And Stripi, who I didn't know.

Monday 23 May.
For happiness you need freedom, and for freedom you need courage.

DEPRA

So said Janez Janša[5] on the radio yesterday. Happiness needs much more than just freedom: school, a job, a future. And as little of the past as possible. It seems to me that the last six months have just been a dream and that I'm living in a time between two wars. People are unhappy. They want bread and circuses. Bread they have to sort out for themselves, while the circuses have been a little gruesome of late. Human life isn't worth much any more. I don't understand. *I don't understand.* The world is rushing headlong into new systems that will allow even faster development, but to what end? Where are we headed? And how long will it take? A lot of us can't handle this pace, many people will become worn out. When the situation's like that, there's not much left. Suffer and make the best of this moral and material confusion ruling us. Chaos. I'm thinking about the end of the world and everything just seems, to put it mildly, ridiculous. All these wars and excuses for industrial, technological, and of course actual exploitation of the undeveloped world. The new-age colonisers have become established. And the new-age crusaders. *I don't understand.* I'm doing ok today. And I'm writing. My psychiatrist said I should write as much as possible. Looks like everything's cool.

So one Monday we came to an evening break.
And a nap, which might come now.
Or maybe not.
Who knows?

---

[5] Prime Minister of Slovenia.

Renata Ažman

Not me.

I've been invited to Israel. Right now I don't dare leave the flat, let alone go to the airport, get on a plane, out, among people. I'm paralysed by fear ... .

God, please, give me a few years without depression, without fear. I deserve it. Please.

Tuesday 24 May.

Today's a quiet day. Today I've been thinking a lot about how important it is to accept my own mistakes, and those of others. Nobody's perfect, and nobody's completely bad. We're all somewhere in between, spread out along a Gaussian curve, sometimes so, other times different. We all have our crosses to bear, and everybody makes mistakes. **Everybody**. So there's no perfect marriage, no perfect union, and no perfect people. Anyone who thinks so is psychotic and should seek immediate help from the nearest psychiatric clinic.
Today's a quiet day. I still can't go out. Luckily I found another packet of old, dried-out cigarettes, in a drawer. Beggars can't be choosers. The smart thing to do would be to stop. But I can't. I don't know how. It's not just my health, it's also my current financial situation. In any event, it's a bad idea for me to spend most of my money on cigarettes. But I just can't help it. It's probably the

DEPRA

same for all smokers. Even if you've got no money for food, there has to be money for cigarettes. *I feel free.* Good morning.

The last time I was at my psychiatrist, I told her that I smoke grass because it helps me work; if I can work, I can earn; if I can earn, I can live. I just told her. And of course she advised me against it. But then she told me I should decide for myself, and of course she'll still help me if she can. Thanks. *Merci.*

I should follow the example of animals. Animals aren't so self-destructive, they don't suffer from depression and they don't have to smoke grass. Animals always know who will lead the pack, who will give birth, who will go hunting and who will laze about. And they don't make a fuss about it. But we're always dramatising. We're always moaning and complaining, and then we wonder why we're all on the verge of madness. Psychiatrists have never been as busy as they are now. I'm always convinced of that when I go. I filed a text. It's an amazing feeling. When you write an article and send it, you don't have to do anything for a while. Or when you know you've got plenty of time and you can do what makes you happy. If anything does. When I'm depressed, nothing cheers me up. I'm still happiest in the evening, when I can finally go to sleep. *Sleep.*

Renata Ažman

Wednesday 25 May

Today used to be a holiday. Tito's birthday, the day of youth. We used to go on a trip, or have a sports day. Now it's just another day.

What will I be, where will I go? I don't know. I'm unbearably afraid.

It's worst in the morning, when you open your eyes and you realise there's another day ahead. But it's not so bad now: it was worse a few years ago. Things were terrible then. Nothing was real anymore, I had nothing to lean on, there was nothing but a world without sense around me. And fear, mindless fear and panic. This went on for years, and it tortured me. I couldn't leave the flat for six months. When I finally plucked up the courage, it was the worst twenty minutes of my life. I was afraid of the pavement I walked on, of passers-by, of the cat crossing the road. I watched the ground, my mind was falling apart from the horror I felt in my bones. At the shop counter, my vision clouded over, shivers ran down my spine, I didn't know who or where I was. Panic attack. When I got back out into the fresh air, it was a little better. Those six months were terrible. But it was like that beforehand, and afterwards. I wouldn't go through that again, no thanks. I've had enough fear for one lifetime.

DEPRA

And I hope that my soul will rest soon, even if it only happens once my earthly life is over. Even then, as long as it's soon. Please.

I find the world becoming more and more like a global Babylon, where you have to know as many foreign languages as possible to survive. My English is quite good, I understand German although I don't speak it, but I'm best at Croatian. But in a way I was born with it, so I don't count it as a foreign language. I'd get by in a foreign country. Recently I read a few pages from an English book. But then I moved and I lost the book, but I know it was about madness. About manic-depressive psychosis. It was written by Jason Pegler, who has the disease himself. What causes madness? Madness is caused by inappropriate patterns we carry in ourselves. And until we overcome them, some of us are sometimes a little mixed up. Sometimes. Some of us. A little. Mixed up.

I was talking to a guy I was in the mental hospital with. He tells me he's not doing too well, he's scared he's going to lose his job when they find out he's being treated by a psychiatrist. Maybe. Everything is possible. Isn't it?

Thursday 26 May

Early this morning, I didn't think I could make it through the day. When I opened my eyes, I was first of all scared by the morning. Then I looked in the mirror and then I realised my fridge was empty. I went to the shop with my last ounce of strength and bought the essentials. Passers-by scared me, as did the shop assistant. There's a black hole in my chest, and every minute it's sucking up all the atoms of my strength, leaving me alone and terrified. Instead of lunch, I'm throwing up. I can't take it any more. I want to die, but I don't have to. I'm already dead.

Friday 27 May

Nothing.

Saturday 28 May

This morning there was a gentle tap on my window, and when I woke, it seemed that the water was gently carrying me down a channel. Finally, it's all the same to me. *Que sera, sera*. For a long time, I've needed to decide to jump from the cliff into the water. Until I realised that there's no point fighting against fate. Wherever it takes me, it will take me. Everything I have and everything I need is packed in my heart, and I hope the angels are watching over me. Before, I was holding on to the bank, and I don't know why. Now I want to swim, let the current take me, let God's will be done. Years ago I visited a fortune-teller who told me everything that then happened. That gave me courage to dare to believe. And she said that I would live

DEPRA

abroad. What is abroad? Sometimes in another country you meet people who are closer than your neighbours and family. National borders cannot stop the searching and yearning. I could of course shut myself up inside my four walls and stare at the title deeds, happy that my plot of land is one square metre bigger than my neighbour's. Everything's allowed. *It's a free country.* Every time I watch the news, I get a little shiver. Accidents, murders, war and politics. So usually I don't even switch the television on. When I'm in a crisis, I just can't watch it. I can't stand it. *Of course.* Every time I think like this about the enigmas of our earthly life, at some point I'm transported into space. I can't understand how an ordinary amoeba can evolve into a mind like the human mind. It has a genius, good and bad. And, wherever you turn, thanks to his brain, man has dominated the Earth and now wants to dominate space as well. But he won't. It seems abundantly clear to me that sooner or later we will encounter another form of life: I can't believe life evolved only on Earth. But I don't understand why we're so very afraid of the prospect. We may encounter friendly beings who will help us. And we really need help. At least Western, white civilisation has become completely devalued by its mindless consumerism. When everything degenerates to the absurd, it's inevitably followed by a painful catharsis and then finally redemption. But this can take hundreds of years. Like it took millions of years for one amoeba to evolve into the lizard, and another amoeba into man.

Renata Ažman

Evolution

I don't believe unconditionally in evolution. It's perfectly possible that the story of Adam and Eve is true. Perfectly possible. *Everything is possible*. So we shouldn't ignore any theory of the beginning and end of the world. In a way, we will never know what actually happened millions of years ago on Earth. All of it is just supposition. We will have to face the simple truth that there are ever multiple realities in the world, and it's increasingly difficult to achieve a consensus among them. *Good thing there's only one God.* Years ago I used to love reading the exciting details of unexplained phenomena, such as crop circles and the interesting measurements of the pyramid of Khufu. Signs, symbols, occult. Now I've got some evidence that there absolutely are other realities, not just the one we call normal. The human mind is limitless, but not unique. Every ant has its own reality, and every elephant, and every bird in the sky. How can we then say that some are normal, and others not? Do you really have to have a house, two kids, a VW Golf and a golden retriever for people to leave you alone? If everything is God's will, then *everything* is God's will: lunatics, prostitutes, gays and tramps, all of it. We can't go half way and only talk of God when it suits us in context. If there is a God, then there is one God for all, and amen. What we call him is up to him. Sometimes people had many gods, like the ancient Greeks and Romans, and later also us, the Slavs. Pagans. I don't know which is better, to worship one god, or to personify and divide God's will

into areas: war god, love god, sea god, sun god. I don't know; seems to me that there is only one God, and I pray to him when I ask for something. God is endless love and energy, filling you with white light and giving you a feeling of security. That's how it looks from my perspective.
God recognises all truths, including that there is no god.

Each of us spreads the word of God in our own way. You see?

End of the world. Still Saturday.

When I'm depressed, everything is hard and black and I ponder death and the end of the world. When I'm in a good mood, I think of life and beginnings and happy endings. So I'm living a double dream. One is more of a nightmare, the other is joyful and beautiful. But why don't we all live that way? With my illness, everything is more explicit. Extreme lows and highs, both of them verging on madness. What is madness anyway? An outburst of the unconscious, the collapse of the existing system and the construction of a new one. If you manage. Once you've been mad, you'll never be normal again. And not just because psychiatrists will brand you as such for ever, but also because the old reality can't be fixed, and the new reality – madness – cannot be denied. The logic of madness is the logic of the unconscious. And if there's something wrong in the unconscious, madness shows it up. In madness you can resolve your greatest traumas, or you may never solve anything and live on ... until the next madness. My resolution of traumas and problems happened *per partes*, in parts. It was all very intense, and now, when I look back at everything that went through my mind, I'm horrified. But evidently, it had to be that way, and God helped me. But not just him. An angel also helped me. An angel, right here on Earth. Me and my soul. Thanks.

Holy angel, guardian mine, be with me always, stand by me night and day, protect me from all that is bad, I humbly beg you, guide me and watch over me. Amen.

Sometimes life seems so complicated, but it's basically so simple. Some people you love without even knowing why. Others you don't like, again without knowing why.
I spoke to Niveska. She's off to the seaside, and is happily packing. She's going to the coast for three months. She's already happy that she'll be on a boat with her son. She tells me she took part in a procession in front of Cologne Cathedral. And she's made her peace with God. It was a Croatian procession and she felt like she was in Zagreb. They even had two flags. We were talking about the beach, the weather (36 degrees in the shade in Cologne!), Nina, the sea and Murvica. I won't see her this year, or maybe ever. So it goes. The Croatian coast is beautiful ... this year I'll only see it on television. Or I'll close my eyes and listen to the rumbling splashing on the rocks, where my

DEPRA

wounded soul has rested so often. I know how the sea whispers, and how it roars. The sea is beautiful everywhere; although I think the Croatian coast is the most beautiful. If everything goes well, I'll be able to make it in the autumn. Maybe not, though. The sea is beautiful everywhere.

In Tel Aviv there's a long stretch of sandy beach, ten, a hundred times longer than the ones I'm used to. And when you walk on the sand, barefoot in the middle of December, you realise that everything is relative.

It seems my life will end somewhere in a very modest forest hut, alone, with my laptop in my arms. Tapping away on the keyboard, assuming of course there's electricity. If not, I'll write in pencil by candlelight. Even more romantic.
Can't have one without the other.
I still best believe old Ančka, who once – more than thirty years ago – told me that I would make my living by writing. And I'd die at 54 in a plane crash, she said. That would be cool. No old age, just boom and it's all over. If I don't get tired of it all before then. I can hang a rope from a door, no problem. I even tried it once, and almost choked. Ha ha ha. *Hm.* Maybe it's not funny. I can't help it, even I have my defence mechanisms; laughter for one. And fear. And drugs. I realise this, and until things change, that's the way it'll be. Amen. It's my life and my account.

Renata Ažman

Sunday, 29 May.

In the last two years I've discovered a number of new worlds, helping me to establish a distance from the reality that I should live in, but never have. Sometimes you just have to believe you're doing the right thing, even if it's not what the people all around you are doing. Sometimes you just have to be different. No choice. Then you meet someone like yourself. Sooner or later. Or do you sit unhappily in a cage of normality, waiting for the end? Which is better? We're not all normal. Some of us are mentally ill. Sorry. Today I was in old Ljubljana; I went with a friend for a late afternoon walk, ice cream and coffee. Two coffees. People were buzzing around, and I felt like I was from another planet. My reality consists of coffee, cigarettes, my keyboard and the phone. And a crate of apples on the balcony. I'm not interested in the things that are the centre of the world for normal people. I look skywards, searching for a sign of the final truth. *Am I mixed up again?*
Why are you writing this book, someone asked the other day. Because someone will read it, and because I love writing. Maybe it will help someone, or help me. I don't know. I've no idea where my therapy ends and yours begins. This life is just one long therapy. We constantly solve some problem and trauma, and worry about right and wrong, and who said what and such nonsense. Bullshit. That's not it. That's not real life. But it's the only one we have here on Earth. And I think it'll

never get any better. The times they are a changing, usually for the worse. So what am I supposed to be happy about?

God help me.

There is one thing, though, that could save this world from collapse. Childish logic. Sometimes it can be really useful to talk to children, as they can lead you to simple understandings just like that, in passing. Generally speaking, I think we should listen to children more. And not take them so lightly. Children know more than we realise. In fact, we should introduce child police, who would discover irregularities and punish offenders. Just to see.

This world is falling apart. A new anthill will emerge from its ruins, with new values, a new world. A new world. And I'm sad I won't be there to see it. It will be beautiful. All new worlds are beautiful to start with.

Without a doubt, there is some system by which our universe operates. Fragments of understanding are given to us in this life, but the essence of the system of the universe, well, only God knows that. God, who sees everything, and knows everything. So it's smart to talk to him, and swap information from time to time. Sometimes something terrible has to happen for you to turn to God. Until then, earthly bonds are enough. But when things are really bad, only God can provide consolation. Always. You just have to open up your heart and believe. Some people don't believe in God, they think it's just nonsense. I thought so too, once. But it's not, at least not in my experience. I've never seen him, but I feel his presence. With every step, and all the time.

"... sleep tight and sweet dreams ..."

I think our basic mission is to love ourselves, and be friendly. If we all worked towards that, and strived for peace and coexistence among people of different cultures, this world would be a very different place. Instead we worry about who's superior, and who's inferior, and it's basically our pride that leads us to think like that. Why should white people be worth more than black people? Or straight more than gay? Or the rich more than the poor? There's no theory to support such attitudes. But in practice? That's a different story.

... it's hard for me to travel, to say goodbye to you ... all the faithless and all the crosses, when you're not here, they're all closer ... I leave my soul to you ...

I want to find a little space on this Earth, a place where I could die in peace. I'd drag myself into a cold cave with a bottle of vodka in the middle of December, and sleep soundly, shaking in the coming day. I've experienced many beautiful things, and even more bad things, but if I believe in God, I also have to believe that it was all God's will. I don't know why I've been thinking about death so much recently; maybe because I'm beginning to have enough of this life. I want to sleep on a little white cloud up in the sky, and only wake up when I'm truly rested. I'm tired. Tired of everything. Everybody wants to die at some point. Sometimes things get complicated and sometimes the idea of dying can save us, help us to live. Catch 22. They're playing a rock version of the *Zdravjica*[6] on the radio. It's funny, our national anthem. It promotes alcoholism, which in my view is one of the biggest problems in this country. And if grass is banned, they should also ban alcohol. I think they're similar, except the effects of alcohol are much more damaging. Alcohol makes you brave and recklessness can have terrible consequences.

Sunday (still).

Tiča called. She's getting on her bike and coming to Ig. I'm pleased. I hope she'll be careful on Ižanka, which can be really dangerous for cyclists. It's too narrow, and two cars and a bike can only pass with difficulty. But it looks like they'll repair the road to Škofljica. It's a better road, because it's shorter and not as dangerous as Ižanka. If I manage to earn enough money in winter for heating, maybe I'll stay here, in Ig. In fact, I very much want to, because I love this flat and this view, which ends somewhere on Krim, and from there

---

[6] The Slovenian national anthem, a poem by France Prešeren.

Renata Ažman

straight towards the sky. Up there are little clouds, my friends, and it calms me. Sometimes in the clouds I find an answer to a question that's been rattling round my brain. Other times, I just watch the clouds dance, scattering creamy lumps here and there.
And it seems more and more to me that I want to go there. Sometime soon. Sometime very soon.
Today was a funny day. Bright and sunny, and all day I've been thinking about death.
Death seems beautiful to me. At least for the person dying; It's harder for those left behind. I know quite a few people who never recovered after losing someone close.

And then you look to the stars and you think he's there. But who?

The sky above Krim is red today. Tomorrow's going to be another hot day. It's becoming less and less clear to me how and why. But I don't bother about that. I'll be alright somehow, Oliver is in good hands. It could all also end up at the psychiatric clinic, easily. Wouldn't be the first time. There's no bogeyman there, if truth be told. The staff are friendly, even the doctors. The only uncomfortable feeling is that you've given yourself up to their mercy, or lack of it.

... but now another loves you, gulps down your eyes ... and I have lost you, my golden one ...

DEPRA

At the clinic, you're basically a person without rights. As soon as you enter the closed ward, everything you say is questioned, every raised voice a sign of aggression, or even psychosis. Inside, you have nothing, not even reality. Your reality is bed, toilet, shower, bright blue pyjamas, and the coffee machine at the end of the corridor. How are you supposed to learn to live again in such an environment? And then you get out. It's not written on your forehead, but everybody knows you've been in the mental hospital. And they start treating you differently. And you don't understand anything. It's as if something important has changed, forever. And then you realise that something inside you died.

Monday, 30 May.

Today I woke up with the familiar feeling of fear in my bones. But I'm not going to get upset. It'll pass. But it is extremely unpleasant. Without any will, I wander around the flat, I want to clean but I drop the duster and go and cry. Now I know this shit will never end. I don't care. I'm not so frightened now, although I want to feel better again as soon as possible. Everything seems pointless. *Really*. Depression is its own reality, unpredictable and treacherous. It sneaks up on you and grabs you round the neck like a python trying to suffocate you. Suddenly the meaning of everything changes, and everything you think of is black.

Renata Ažman

God help me.

This is basically my last attempt to say that I'm in a bad way, and I don't want to be. But I am, and then some. I don't know how things will turn out, and I don't care. I'm not afraid to die. That's the only important thing. Maybe I'll start to become scared of it later, I don't know. But for now, I'm more afraid of living than dying.

God, please, take me to you. I don't like it here; it's hard.

Tuesday, 31 May.

It's raining outside and I can scarcely see Krim because of the fog. If you look long enough in the same direction, you can see the blurry outline of a green slope, rising powerfully from the grassy plains of the Ljubljana marsh. I'm privileged to live in a national park, and I hope that I don't have to leave this flat for money reasons. A colleague told me yesterday that years ago she wrote an article on marijuana, and one of the things she discovered is that it's even used as a treatment for depression in certain hospitals in England. She promised she'd find the article so that I can read it. I'd be very interested. I don't know about anyone else, but it helps me. *Today is World No Tobacco Day. And I haven't got any cigarettes. Outrageous.* I can hear the raindrops hitting the tops of the trees and spraying my

window. A spring storm is something wonderful. And the bushes. *God is angry.*
I'm not going to the coast this year. I'll stay at home with my computer and write. I think it might well help someone with the same illness as me, so that they no longer feel so isolated just because they're not normal. When I took Japajade[7] to my psychiatrist to read, she said to me: "Renata, you don't even need me. Next time you're depressed, just read your book." I took that as a great compliment, and I can only hope that the book will really help someone make it through a difficult patch.

Depression passes.
Sometimes it's enough just to know that you're not the only one, not alone in your unhappiness. It helped me a great deal. After long, painful years, when I raised my head from the sand and recognised some home truths and facts, I was better. I recommend the same for you, if you're suffering from depression. I've also been helped by one simple fact that we must keep in mind all the time: depression passes. Fears leave. *Whenever.* Of course, when you're on the ground and you're beating yourself up for God alone knows what delusion, it's hard to believe that it will pass. That it will ever pass. The worst thing is when you know very well what you're doing is wrong, but you can't help it. It's wrong – so the doctors say – to lie around in bed and sleep. But when I'm depressed, that's exactly what I do. Now at

---

[7] Japajade, the author's first book.

least I don't have a guilty conscience about it; sometimes I couldn't forgive myself for being so useless. And then that was killing me too. I can still remember exactly how it all began. I woke up one morning in a mindless fear. I went straight from sleep to a panic attack, which didn't and wouldn't ease up. It went on for months, finally culminating in manic psychosis, which was why I ended up in Polje[8] for the first time. The second time – again after a long and painful period of depression – I ended up on Brač, and went to a psychiatrist in Split. Third time, back to Polje. For three weeks. Maybe I'll have to go into hospital again, but I'm not afraid of it any more. Or rather, I want not to be afraid. I put on a brave face to myself and to others, but inside there's a weak child who more than anything else in the world wants a warm and safe refuge, like any child. There's just such a child in each of us, and we must love it unconditionally and listen to it, since it leads us to inner transformation, through cathartic minutes hidden in moments of meditation and conversations with God. Whenever we ask about the fundamentals, it's a good idea to know the answer in advance, although it never happens and in life you have to be reckless often so that you can learn from your mistakes. Some of these lessons are damned expensive and you wind up asking yourself: why me? The answer is not straightforward, and it's hard to justify. Fate? God's will? Karma? Accident? I don't know. I do though remember that I always believed everything

---

[8] Ljubljana Psychiatric Clinic

DEPRA

would work out in the end. But then the question arose, when the end would be. When would the period predicted by all the fortune tellers I've ever visited start? Each and every one of them found a great deal of happiness in the end in the various signs of my future. But I'm still depressed; still broke; and in the evening I pray to fall asleep and close my eyes against the black shadows climbing into my soul. Only faith in God can exorcise them, and I'll have to recognise that.

Last day of May.

Today it feels like I've lopped one head off the dragon. How many heads are left? Just when I think I've cut off the last, two new ones appear. *I'm alone.* Like a tramp from Tromostovje[9]. When I was at secondary school, I spent some time with tramps. One summer we met up and at the time it still wasn't clear to me what it's like to be homeless. In the evening we would sit together in Zvezda and smoke grass, then I would catch the last bus home, while they ... well I never asked where they went. Only later, one winter after Zlatko had frozen to death and he just wasn't around any more in the spring, did I think about it. They slept under bridges and in the dark doorways of Old Ljubljana. It was possible back then, but now more and more of the doorways are locked up.

Everybody's afraid of tramps. But they're just people too.

---

[9] A well-known hangout for homeless people in Ljubljana.

Renata Ažman

I don't know the words I have to write, all I know is that they'll be *those* words, as a consequence of which I'm now sitting in front of my computer with my eyes closed, trying to drag them out of the babble of memories and people involved in my life in one way or another. Making peace with God means making peace with yourself, with your virtues and your mistakes, accepting everything that life brings, good or bad. I don't know just how much one person can take, but judging from my own experience, it's a lot.

God never burdens you with more than you can bear. My life has entered the second half, and all that I can do is not repeat the same old mistakes. Enjoy myself and slowly but surely withdraw from this stage, on which the young, healthy, beautiful and gifted are already arriving. Beginnings are always beautiful. When I stood alone on the verge of a career in journalism, I was into everything, everything was new and exciting. Now it seems like it was all a single moment, trapped in time and space, and I supped from the fountain with the wrong spoon. But I didn't have any other. Then my health packed in and the dragon arrived. Like that guy in The Fisher King. But then I fought; sometimes I would lie in bed in the evening, exhausted, hoping I'd die in my sleep. Then the dragon started appearing in my dreams, and there was no safe haven for me in this world. But I still fought. Now I don't care, even though it's eating me up. I'm not afraid any more. No, it's more than that. I want it to consume

me and destroy me once and for all, so that this farce will finally come to an end. Chicken run. Life is like a chicken run. Short and shitty. For a long time I've been trying to live, rushing along this dusty road, even though I've no idea where it's heading. I just hope it'll all be over at some point. I'm surrounded by desert, wandering without water but with hope in my heart. *Is that normal?*
It's still raining. The freshened sky smells of ozone and the plants are gratefully turning towards the sky. The cats in the courtyard are looking for shelter beneath cars; the sparrows and titmice are monitoring the situation from beneath projecting roofs. Today's the last day of May and tomorrow it's June already. I can't believe how quickly time's passed.

June 2005.

This year May was hot and sunny, but June turned out to be wet. On the fifteenth, I handed in the corrections to the Japajade manuscript. When I got home, I lay down on the couch, closed my eyes and resolved from that point on to leave everything to God. I can't take it any more. I'll write as long as I can, and then ... then I don't know. Tomorrow that nice teacher's coming to view the flat again, maybe she'll buy it; I'm moving into a smaller and cheaper flat.
I don't need 90 square metres. And I'm repaying a loan.
What sort of world would I want to live in? Different from the one I'm living in now. Just and fair. Friendly

Renata Ažman

to children and animals. People would be friendly to each other, and the demons would be dead before they're even born. Obviously this world is the Kingdom of God on the one hand, and the devil's realm on the other, a world in which from time to time all the darkest and most horrible features of human nature emerge: bullying, child abuse, cruelty to animals, torture – physical or mental – and hatred for anyone different. Those – in my humble opinion – are the five modern deadly sins, which could easily be added to those so colourfully portrayed by David Fincher in the unforgettable film Seven. *Seven*. Today's another one of those days when I just want to die. I'd like to lie in bed, cover my head and let my soul float away, to the New World.

In the New World, everything's ok: no rows, no plotting and intrigue, no money or other material goods. Love rules there.

The Earth is a polygon on which at every step you encounter Good and Evil. Sometimes the former wins, and sometimes the latter. And so Earth is dominated by a wide range of good works, mixed up with an even more diverse collection of crimes, many of them unpunished. Those who believe in justice are most often disappointed, as are those who swear by honesty and sincerity. Even proverbs urge people not to be good. *Good deeds go unrewarded. It doesn't pay to be good.* And so on, as if we've already quietly legitimised

DEPRA

lies, deception, greed and scheming. That's not good. The problem is, people generally think that beauty lies in money and material pleasures. The poor souls don't realise that the greatest beauty is hidden in the soul open to Love that talks to God. It's only possible if you're sincere and ready for anything. Even for death, which one day will come knocking to rescue you from living on the polygon of life and suffering, which in one form or another everyone on Earth experiences. In the New World there's no suffering. No pain, no fear. In the New World, all those who come are children. Small, playful, happy children. In the New World, everything is ... *completely different.*

The basic problem with this world is that stupid people have children. To have a child is an act of responsibility. So anyone who wants children should be tested to see if they're up to the responsibility. Often, a couple will only decide – under pressure – to live together when there's a baby on the way. How can a child in such circumstances grow up to be a normal person? Arguments, violence and other misfortunes that happen to children stem from that simple fact: the wrong people have children. While we have nothing. Good thing I believe in the New World; otherwise, I don't know how it would be.

I die again every day. Where are you, New World?

Renata Ažman

Still June 2005.
I was in a shop when I saw her ... a little girl in a green top with a ribbon in her hair. She was all alone in the middle of her mother's favourite supermarket. In her excessive shopping frenzy, her mother had lost her. The little girl found herself alone amid the giant boxes of conditioner and cheap washing powder. Suddenly there were no more familiar faces, hands she so liked to hold, the buggy in which her baby rucksack was resting. She was turning in circles, abject terror spreading to her soul. Then, holding her teddy bear tightly in her arms, she stepped bravely into the unknown. So she walked, and people were bumping into her, when she saw the door. She went out, into the air, but she still didn't know where she was, or where her mummy was. I found her terrified in front of the big shop. She was crouching in the corner by the exit, hugging her teddy bear and crying.
"What happened?" I asked her.
"Mummy, where's my mummy ..."
"What's your name?"
"Malusa"
"Well Maruša, let's go find your mummy." She took my hand and we set off towards the counter with the large hanging Information sign. I asked the lady behind the counter to page little Maruša's mum over the PA. She did so, and in just a few minutes Maruša's mum turned up at the counter. The child, happy to have found her lost treasure, fell into her arms. And what did her mum do? She gave her a slap.

DEPRA

"Why did you get lost?" her mum shouted. No hug, no commiseration, just anger. I felt I should say something, but I didn't. *God forgive me. I should have done.*

In the maze. Still June.
We're all sometimes lost little girls like Maruša. Lost in a horrible maze of problems, and we can't see an end, or a beginning, or any solutions. Sometimes we're to blame for our own problems. Not always though. There are subjective and objective problems. One objective problem for instance is an economic crisis. A crisis of values. System collapse. Existence, illness, disappointment. Faced with problems like these, we're more or less on our own. More or less, because at the bottom of my heart I still believe it isn't so. But every day, I persuade myself again that it is. But what can I do? I'm too small to change the world. The only thing I can do is change myself. But why? I want to die, and I've had enough. So I don't care. I've laid my life at God's feet for him to do as he will. I can't take any more. I don't know how.
For people like that, it's best we die.
I don't care. I can't look for doors anymore, not when I probably won't ever find any. Maruša's still a child. She has everything in front of her. I don't know if that's a blessing or a curse. The paradox of this world is they learn one thing and do another. On television recently we've been hearing ever more carefully formulated and contrived statements. Nobody's being honest, telling us

Renata Ažman

what the situation is and what's really important. We live in a chaotic world of nothing and false promises, and that can't be good. There are a few – very influential – people among us for whom such a situation is ideal. The rest of us try to find our way through the system. We think we're doing ok. Nobody considers that we've already long since crossed the line of decent living. The events we're living through show us every day that we're trapped in a loop created for us by others. It's all the same to me, I just want to die. But those of you with children should care what sort of world they'll live in. Starting at the beginning, we should stop all wars. Armies should be disbanded, and disputes resolved in court. The human system is designed to be paranoid, so that we have to defend or attack. Even in the name of God. We should conserve nature. But most of all we should respect others, and those different from us. Black and white, white and black first of all. Then more: women men, and men women – and both of them their children. More and more it seems that my New World is a rambling utopia. Even so, I won't stop believing in it – it's the last thing I've got left.

Don't cry, my love, what was last night,
your hand comforts me, I must leave at dawn
... I dream of freedom for you, so don't cry ...
and when the last sun spreads, when the yellow flower blooms,
a scream builds in my throat, I'm not sad to be dying ...

DEPRA

guide me, try me, when freedom is my sin,
be peaceful in my soul ... when I stand before the wall.

White bears. Still June.
I'd like to see polar bears up close one time. I'd *really* like to. Maybe they're wild. But it sometimes feels like I could get on more easily with them than with some people. Such is our crazy world: telecommunications miracles, but no communication. This world is ripe for a total transformation. Perhaps now, when I'm in depression, I see everything to be darker than it really is. I don't know. I do know though that I've never felt really good in this world. I liked it best in the forest, away from people. All my fairy tale heroes lived in the forest. Maybe that's why the forest was so often my last refuge. I'd lie down under a tree and watch the leaves dancing in the wind. The only noise would be the rustling of dried leaves on the ground, and the odd branch. Otherwise, they were moments of silence and peace, the perfection of which I've never found anywhere else in the world. I would play in a hill stream with Ada, a German mastiff, who would fetch sticks; those were my happy moments. *Happy only then.*

Today the forests are different, or maybe it just feels that way. In the beauty spots, people swarm in loud tracksuits, looking for their little piece of blue sky. But it's not like that any more. You can't rest in peace under a tree and dream. They disturb you. Deep in the old forest, you might still find such peace, but I can't. If I

Renata Ažman

close my eyes I can find myself right under that pine tree where I so often lay, thinking about the future. About God, if he exists. They never told me about him.

To sleep, perchance to dream. So said Hamlet. Was he also depressed?

DEPRA

Moving.
It looks like I've sold the flat. It seems that the rhyming advert helped. The friendly estate agent suggested I write it myself, so I did: "In the middle of a grassy plain, in the heart of the Ljubljana marsh nature reserve, stands a house with six flats. The one for sale is on the first floor, cool in summer and warm in winter, where I love to live, waking in the morning and going to sleep in the evening to a wonderful view of Krim. Three rooms, kitchen, bathroom, WC, pantry, large balcony, cellar, garage, pleasant surroundings and friendly people. Far from the hustle and bustle of the city, but close enough to the centre of Ljubljana that you won't feel cut off from the world. And in the evening, when the only sound is made by the crickets in the grass, the sun bids you good night from behind Krim." A friendly teacher, who liked the advert, fell in love with the flat a few days later and if it all goes according to plan, she'll buy it. I'm so pleased. It's not easy to sell such a big flat in Ig these days. I really want to know what sort of flat I'll find. My den. I can hardly wait. I'll furnish it the way I've always wanted. I'll find it myself. They say that moving house is like your house burning down. Moving to me seems an ideal opportunity to get rid of things I don't need. It's just getting ready takes a while. I'll need to go to the shops for boxes: one at a time, but I'll get there.
I know the drill. I can't move! But I have to.
I'm fine, because I've got somewhere to go. What about the thousands and thousands of people who pay high

rents for a room or a flat, and will never have the chance to experience the joy of a home of their own? Or those who've worked hard and saved and built all their lives, and what do they have to show for it? A house that needs heating, windows that need replaced, a yard that needs sweeping. And a low wage or a pension that's barely enough for the essentials. The tragedy of the modern age is that people who ten years ago were comfortable are being slowly reduced to poverty. Poverty in Slovenia is hidden behind thick walls, in which many have invested money and energy all their lives, but suddenly find there's nothing they can do with them. The lucky ones have parents who can help them get their own flat. And lottery winners. What about the rest? The homeless and the unemployed? Park benches are fine in the summer ... what about in the winter?

... I'll sell the skirt,
for a little sweet wine,
I'm not, not, not going home,
I'm too thirsty.

Mad world. Still June.

Something wonderful happened. The teacher who, so it seems, will buy my flat, totally surprised me. When we met for the second time in our lives and we'd only just started to be less formal, our conversation turned to food. I said that I didn't have much because I had no money. And the lady stood up and went to the shop,

DEPRA

coming back with two stuffed shopping bags, including a carton of cigarettes. Taken aback, I thanked her and she said that someone else had done the same for her, and that it's a tradition that should be encouraged. *Cool.* I've started packing. All signs are that I've sold the flat.

It's hard to come to terms with the fact that everything that's happened in my life happened according to God's will. I don't know why I had to go through such hard times, but somewhere in the end ... *in young birches a silent spring, in young birches dreams nesting* ... I'll have an answer to this question. ... *for all those big and small who still believe in it.*
I remember as a little girl I was always visiting my neighbour's dog. I would snuggle up beside him, and he kept me warm and safe. He was called Ringo and I was very sad one day when he was no longer in the yard. I never found out what happened to him. *He was my friend and solace. I felt safe in his fur.* I can't go on. My brain no longer perceives the reality I'm used to, and I'm seriously worried about whether I can even live in this mad world. *Probably not.* I'm becoming completely apathetic; still, it's better than depression. Depression is a devil eating away at your soul little by little, drinking and drinking like it will never stop. Once I was so tired after working all day that I fell asleep in the hall, still wearing my coat and shoes. I just collapsed as soon as I got home. I woke up the next morning, sore everywhere. Outside and in. I don't want to go back to

those times. But even now it's not easy. For me or with me. Is it?

New world. Still June.
The golden bird is singing to me. Only I can understand her song, she's singing to me.
Good thoughts and kind deeds. That's the New World.
I'm sitting by the window, listening. The wind is catching the treetops as if it wants to pull them out by the roots. The golden bird is silent. And that was all it had to say.

Fear. July 2005.

It's the middle of summer, and I'm still in a deep depression. I can't go out.
On a shelf in the room are two packets of 0.5 milligram Xanax and my usual pills. And an envelope with a referral to Polje. All options are still open and ... I'm afraid.
I don't want to be afraid. But I don't know how much longer.
They're coming again, the fears, the dragon and all that remains of this, my earthly life. I hope that I'll be going to the next world soon. If it all gets too much, I'll gather my strength and ... no, I won't kill myself. I don't have the courage. And sometimes I really like being alive. Maybe for an hour a day. Shit, why haven't they invented a painless suicide pill. They should sell it in

DEPRA

pharmacies. I don't understand why our civilisation doesn't let people die when they want to. But if you want to die ... you have to have courage. And I don't. That's why I'm confused. So it goes. Right now I'm in a bad phase, with no money. And no will to work. I'm living in an old one-room flat in Šiška[10], with nothing the way it should be. The fridge is dead, the washing machine jumps, even the computer's got a virus. I'm on the brink of survival, in a dark depression, eased only by ... nothing ... and with a referral to Polje.

Dragon.
I've got nothing in life, nothing except this writing, which at least always reminds me that I'm not a complete loser. Yep, that's depression. Nothingness, surrounded by darkness and an even greater nothingness. A hole in the soul, a hundred-headed dragon that never stops, and that persecutes me when I open my eyes and when I close them in the evening. I want to live like other people, who see and have some sense. But I can't handle it. Every time I start to think about it, or whenever I want to climb a few rungs up the ladder, it drags me back down, so that once again I find myself at the bottom of this well, curled up in a ball, scared out of my wits. This week I decided to try working again. On Monday – today's Wednesday – I was at the Red Cross, and on Thursday – tomorrow – I'm going to Debeli Rtič, where five hundred children from poor families are on holiday. The holiday is

---

[10] A district of Ljubljana.

Renata Ažman

funded by Tuš, a trading company, and when I mentioned this to Alenka, she said that in gratitude for such a gesture she'd shop only in Tuš, if there was a branch near her. But unfortunately there isn't. I'm still ok. God knows what it's like for poor people without even a pension. I hope that I'll manage – if I have to – to survive on 85,000 a month. With my fee of course, which I'm saving for ... I'm not saving anything. It'll be alright. It won't be so expensive to live in this flat, and I'll pick up the odd thing. It's also true that I'm depressed and I see everything even more darkly. It's very hot today. The steam's rising from Celovška and the sun is still mercilessly scorching. I'm not ok, the fear is gnawing at my bones again and doesn't want out. I don't know what will happen, or how I'll be.

I want to die.

I'm having fewer and fewer ideas, my brain is tired from the endless self-doubt, the fight for survival and depression. My spirit has been injured by the lies and chaos ruling this world. There's no justice any more, no systems work like they should, and I think war is coming. It's probably already started, it's just there's not been any official declaration of like there used to be. I know I'm not the only one who's depressed. They say it's very common these days. And the antidepressants are clearly not helping any more. I'll stop fighting, it's the only thing I haven't tried. I'll come to terms with my miserable solitary life, which will last as long as it lasts.

DEPRA

I don't know how and where it will all end, I just hope it's not painful. I'm writing. It's the only thing I know and can do at this fucked-up time. If it gets really bad, I'll go to Polje. They'll take care of me there, or maybe not; what do I know, what do I care? I'll go with the flow – it'll take me where it takes me. I can't go on. I c-a-n'-t go on. To hell with all the positive thoughts I'm trying to bring to mind; to hell with all the good advice I've always been able to give to others; to hell with me. I can't. I can't drag myself out of the sea of unpleasant memories, from the grip of the everyday, with its merciless pressure and endless demands: pay the bills, go to the shops, go out, among people. Where should I go, what should I wear, and how should I get there when I can't even get to the bottom of the stairs? And I've no idea how I'll do that story tomorrow. But I'm going.

I have to go. I'll still be a little scared. God help me.

Jasna came round for coffee. She knows about depression. We said a lot, much more than normal for a half-hour visit. Then she had to go to a press conference. She gave me new courage, and that's part of the reason I'm feeling a little better. I called Saša about Debeli Rtič, but I didn't get her. By now though I should know who's doing the pictures. I'll try again a little later. I hope I can manage a good story. And that I won't be too scared. I called Šent, an association for psychiatric patients. They say they don't give advice over the telephone, but they'll try to find a number for me. And they did. I called, and got Roza. She works on a freephone line, with volunteers available 24 hours a day to talk with you. A real luxury. Thanks, whoever set up the phone line.

SOS. Still July.

I don't know why I didn't call before.
Saša tells me that Manca will be taking pictures tomorrow. Fine.
We arranged to meet at quarter to ten. I talked to Manca on the phone, and asked her to write the story if the whirlwind of despair comes for me overnight and I'm too afraid in the morning to go. She promised she would if she has to; I hope she doesn't. I know she won't have to, because I'll go even if it kills me. It's much easier knowing that I won't have to hide it if I have a panic attack. I don't know if I'm doing the right thing telling everyone what's wrong with me, but that's my therapy. Talking, talking and more talking. An energetic dialogue keeps you going, nothing else. Alone, you're powerless. You're dependent on the energy of others who – fortunately – are still living in this world and are ready to listen. *Connections*. And if God's plan is to be believed, then everything that happens in this world is right. Everything happens for a reason, and everything ends for a reason. So I'll take my life in my hands and try to get out of it what I can. I'm ready again for a fight, however long it takes. I'll

use every available means. I discovered talking on the phone helps. I gain a little energy. Every fifteen minutes. It'll work out. I've been worse.

<u>Totally down.</u>
But what if it's always as bad as the first time? I'll have to learn to live with this. Not easy. But it passes. The worst thing is, while it lasts, you don't think it'll ever stop. It's all in my head, but my head is empty. So? That's the story of my life. Struggling with the illness for every inch of my brain, fighting my fears and struggling for bread. But I won't give up, oh no! Sometimes, though, sometimes it's really bad. Anyone who's had depression knows that. I wouldn't wish it on anybody. Anybody. Sometimes I'd really rather have some other illness, but I guess so does everybody who's ill. Everybody thinks their pain is the worst. And you have to respect pain. I don't know anybody who could say they have a happy life. Everybody's got too much or too little of something or other; everybody. At my age illness is not unusual. The woes of daily capitalist life knock mercilessly on our door, and those who don't succumb are lucky. I don't know what'll happen to me. I'll probably go to hospital for a while after I've filed the report from Debeli Rtič. Unless something else happens. I'm not sure anything else would help me. The lesson for today – it's still Wednesday – is that even joints don't help me much. And I'll run out of them soon enough. I have to stand on my own two feet, nothing helps. Or go to hospital, if nothing else helps.

Renata Ažman

But what happens when you come out again and everything's swarming around you? I could do with a little rest. Definitely. I even managed to write the report. It won't exactly be great, but it seems decent enough. I hope it's published. Today is Saturday, and they say it's going to be hot again. Apparently it was 41 degrees yesterday. This morning I was at the shops, and I wasted 8 thousand. I bought the essentials, the cheapest, and it seems I spent too much. Cigarettes. I can't cope without them. I've stopped making plans; I live from minute to minute. I've resigned myself to my fate. *Que sera, sera*. I've been thinking a lot about God. And wondering what sort of mercy lets all this happen to me. For the first time in ages, I feel like a single person. Before, it always felt there were two of me, with a vicious war between us. War outside, war inside … no wonder I can't do anything. Even writing's hard. Only talking on the phone cheers me up. And it seems to me … oh, nothing. Nothing seems to me. I'm totally down. One way or another.

The end? Still July.

Today is Sunday and miraculously, my soul is at peace. I deserve it. For the moment, the fear has gone, but I'm waiting for the return of my love of life, something I've lost often on this thorny path. God has placed a great burden on me, but it means I'm strong and that I'll slowly dig my way out of the state I'm in. In fact, today I feel good. In a heavenly peace, I'm listening to the Ars

DEPRA

channel – Mozart's on at the moment – and I'm doing fine. I imagine as you read these lines your spirit will be a little easier when you realise that there's still someone in this world fighting the illness – the plague of our century – that we simply call depression. But that's not all. The dragon has many faces, and it's good to find a way to overcome and escape it. I didn't manage. I had to surrender, and it's easier now. Maybe that's the way. You give up, what will be, will be. Of course it's easier for me, because I've not got children or responsibilities, but believe me, sometimes it's actually harder for me for the very same reasons. There's nobody I can devote my life, my time, my love to. That's why I imagine all sorts of things to help me through this life, at times lonely and desolate, at other times joyful and glad.

The inner child. July.
Happy, when I laugh with my inner child. Stroke this child, snuggle up to it and tell it how much you love it. You'll see: your heart will revive, the blood will course through your veins and life will have a meaning you never knew before. Open your heart to your own existence, and indulge yourself. Don't torment yourself with questions and problems that will not get any easier, and may become harder. Don't pay too much attention to money and material possessions, because they won't make you happy. The only thing that can make you happy is love in your heart and honest relationships with the people you love. Don't create a

Renata Ažman

false public image because you think you're not good
enough as you are. That you are the way you are is
God's will, as is everything that happens to you. So
love yourself, and value yourself, and tell yourself
every step of the way that you love yourself. I admit I
don't always manage it too well myself, even though I
know it's the only way. I know. When you're depressed,
you can't love yourself, and nothing helps you escape
the vicious circle of guilt, self-accusation and profound
sadness. When your heart's caught in the net of such
feelings, nothing matters. So when you're in such a
state, it's best to drag yourself off to some corner, calm
down, maybe take a little sedative and wait for it to
pass. Because it will always pass. Sometimes it lasts a
day, sometimes a week, even a year, or two, or more.
But it passes. Sometimes, when it's really bad, even this
insight doesn't help much. But it's still the only thing a
person can rely on at such times. Many people don't
know what it's like when you're depressed. Only those
of us who have been through it really understand it.
And it's hard at the time to put into words the feelings
tearing you apart body and soul. Many people don't
believe you, they think that if you're depressed you're
bluffing, that you can help yourself. And some people
can. Exercise helps some people, but others don't have
the will or the strength for it. They say that sometimes
you have to force yourself, but I've never managed it. I
just ended up feeling worse. Now, finally, a few days
ago, I helped myself with a phone call. And it helps to
tell people what's up with you. If you shut yourself up

DEPRA

in a wall of silence, perhaps even hiding what's happening to you, at some point you end up alone. Maybe not completely alone, but alone, alone in your soul. Not a nice feeling. And don't condemn yourself if you can't work. When you're depressed, every step, any work, takes incredible effort, and if you haven't had depression you simply can't understand. But that's the way it is: I know it, and so probably do you. The worst time is the three weeks waiting for the antidepressants to kick in. Then the only safe place is a corner in your bedroom, or somewhere where nobody will bother you and where you'll have peace. Peace.

Illness.

Depression is a serious illness and you have to act accordingly. If you don't know what it's like, at least try and believe me. Nobody wants to be shoved into this hole with no way out. Many people kill themselves when they're depressed – like two great writers who had this illness, Ernest Hemingway and Virginia Woolf. One shot himself, the other stuffed her coat pockets with stones and walked into a river. One time some psychiatrist – even they are powerless against this illness – told me that only selected people have this illness – manic-depressive psychosis. When I'm depressed, I'd say thanks very much for being chosen, but I'd rather live some other story. But what do we want? Such is life, and we all have our crosses to bear. The sooner you come to terms with your illness, the easier it is. If you fall ill, you're not well; and if you're not well you can't work and you need to see a doctor. Anti-depressants will help you out of the dead end; believe me. So it's smart to take them. I've been taking them for years and I think they help me; without them, the depressive phases would be much, much worse. Today for the first time I stood in front of the mirror and told myself that I'm brave. Then something inside me said "I love you." And I answered "And me you." And that was that. Accept yourself, your appearance, your life. The way things are is the way they're meant to be, and the future, well who knows what the future has in store for us? I don't. I'm glad if my friends are happy. But they're not, most of them anyway. It seems that in the world today there's less and less happiness and more and more other things: fear of illness, fear of unemployment, fear of the unknown. It seems that nobody in the world is completely happy. Everybody has problems and things to do, to solve, to forget. Sometimes it would be really nice if you could just forget the bad things and only remember the good. But that's normal life. Depression is different. When you're depressed, you blame yourself and punish yourself; you think you're a criminal or a worthless nobody. You're not, but when you're depressed you can't think straight.

Sunday. Still July.
Today's break is doing me good. I got a nice pleasant smiley and I can say it's a nice day. Much nicer than before. Thank God for such a day, thanks little angel for the smiley and for the lunch I'm about to eat. I

DEPRA

made rib soup yesterday, and today it will be delicious. I forgot to mention something important: my favourite window flower has a new bloom. If that's not a reason to celebrate, I don't know what is. Last night I took a Xanax, maybe it'll bring me peace. And I hope the peace will last as long as possible. At least so I can write. When things are at their worst, I'm not prepared to sit at the computer. True, I've noticed that my mood swings are getting faster and sharper. It makes me hope that maybe my depression might finally end. Based on my own personal knowledge and experience, it seems that depression is a terrible block on the heart chakra. When I'm depressed I feel anxiety and fear in my chest. Once the fear lifts, I feel fifty kilos lighter. Please God, let the peace last and last and last. Please, pretty please. Will God grant my request? I don't know. I hope so. He's granted so many already.

And I truly hope he'll grant me this one too. Please.

I remember the precise moment when depression hit me for the first time. I was writing my dissertation, working by day and writing at night, and I think that – and all the trauma from my childhood – was the reason I was first attacked by fear. Then I somehow snapped out of it. I took pills for about five weeks, and it passed. I began to go to work, and was satisfied for quite some time. But then I woke up one morning with the dragon squeezing my throat and refusing to let go. I went to the editorial office and told everyone that I was finished,

Renata Ažman

that I was petrified and that I couldn't work. They put me on sick leave; I went back to work after a week, but the fear was still there. I had a very powerful inbuilt feeling of self-criticism, and in the end it almost destroyed me. Now I know where I am. Or at least I no longer bother about who I am and what I am. It's all the same to me. They say there are an awful lot of people with depression in Slovenia lately. No wonder. We're living in difficult times, and each and every one of us faces endless new disasters and obstacles to overcome. It's as if there's no longer any peaceful place to run and hide and wait for it all to go away. When I was at my lowest, I wanted to crawl off to a bear's den, where it would be nice and warm and friendly. Maybe I'm only depressed because I don't know how to write about it. I've read quite a few books about this illness, but unfortunately many of the authors didn't write from experience. I don't know. Maybe I just haven't found the right book. Obviously, many people face difficult trials in life. But depression is a special illness. It changes you permanently. And you learn something from it all. And you meet the angels.

Thank you angels, just for existing. The very fact that there's someone alive in the world that cares about you helps. Contact. Genuine human contact. Thank you God.

It's half three, and I still haven't eaten anything. There's soup in the fridge – work, please, sweetie – and I'm

DEPRA

sure it'll be lovely this evening. Otherwise, I don't cook much. Partly because my kitchen's tiny, partly because I can't face it, and partly because, because ... because I can't face it. I'll eat a piece of bread and dried sausage, drink a little yoghurt. In any event, I need to lose some weight. But I won't. Sorry, but right now I can't afford fruit, vegetables or other healthy food. I buy bread, maybe some yoghurt, milk and butter, the rest I get. T h a n k s.

Angels.
It's muggy out today, but there's a nice breeze coming through the blinds, which I've let down. Today I learnt that I have to help myself, because I'm the only one who can help. I'll learn to live on a pension and I'll write this book. It may never become a book, but so what? Seems to me that depression would interest many people, because people still know too little about this illness. Of course, doctors, psychiatrists, can diagnose you. But how to act when depression appears, that's another question. How to live? You have to use all available means. Without pills, it probably won't work. I don't know. Someone recently asked me if I dared to live as if each day was my last. Do I dare? I'm in a situation where I've got nothing else left. Depression is miserable. Your brain doesn't work, there's just unbearable anxiety and fear. Tomorrow I'm going to switch the electricity and phone to my name. What a hero. Like going to the shops. If you're depressed, these are major achievements. Tomorrow is Monday, the first

of August. It's unusual for a month to start on a Monday. In fact it's rare. I'll try to get through it as best I can, peacefully, stress-free and sensibly, as best I can. Tomorrow I'm going out, then I can do everything else from home. Nothing's going to happen if I go out. But of course, if I'm afraid, I won't go. Just to the shops. I can pay the bills by phone, and I can mail my column. Once a month though I have to go to Slavica to hand over the bills. Shouldn't be a problem. I'll live modestly, like I have been doing, and I'll pray my fridge or washing machine don't pack in. That would be a real blow to my budget. Now Tiča comes. My little angel. And above my bed hangs a real angel, strumming on his angelic guitar and watching over me. Tiča gave me the angel. And it's not the first one she's given me. I've still got one in my treasure chest.

Monday, 1st August.

I'm always a little afraid in the morning, but then I light a cigarette and drink my coffee, and I feel better. I've got to go into town today, so I'm afraid.
And when I try to work out what it is I'm afraid of, I don't have an answer. Everything. But it's not so bad just now. It's often been worse, much worse. In the past, it's often got so bad I couldn't even leave the house. I'd sit for months and months staring at one point trying to find a way out. And then it just happened. I was communicating again, I was working again, and I was ok. But then I'd fall back into a black hole, and again drag myself out. Everybody finds

DEPRA

themselves in a black hole at some point, how deep they know best. And what will my inner voice have to say?

This is your path. Follow it, and enjoy every moment. Don't look back, don't ask what comes next. Walk in peace and seek your dreams. Follow your heart, and God will help you.

Until my first bout of depression, I didn't know my inner voice. Then I read Solomon's book The Meta-Human and I discovered that you have to establish friendly relations with your inner voice. I wanted it to be on my side, a friend. But it wasn't. Nothing was right, nothing was good. It went on for a long time, and I don't know exactly when my inner voice was first on my side. Now it is here, mine, and for me, reliable and friendly. It tells me I'm worth something, that I deserve a little rest and that I should stop taking this life so deadly seriously. Sometimes it would be nice to have a few beers, forget a little and stop worrying about problems that don't exist. But in depression, everything is a problem.

Be strong! When you're standing on the threshold of a new life, you'll be happy. Be patient.

My inner voice sometimes speaks Slovenian, sometimes English.

Renata Ažman

Don't ask why something happened. All of life is God's divine plan and you are part of it. Go with the flow, give in to life. Start to live!

Sometimes I close my eyes, and in my mind, I'm moving to heaven. At such times, many things become clear. People who have died are still alive in my heart. I don't know what happened to their souls, and I also don't know what will happen to ours, but it's a nice feeling, the idea that the memory of someone who has gone can live on. In my mind, I talk to people who I loved and who have died. But not all of them. Only those who never hurt me.

Don't be afraid, it will all be alright. Get ready to be happy. Life has placed many obstacles in your way, and you've overcome them bravely. What you are living through is God's plan, and all that he expects of you is to follow your inner voice. It will tell you where you're coming from, and where this path leads. Good luck!

I spoke to Melita. She says that the text from Debeli Rtič is perfectly clear, and that she's already passed it on. I'm very pleased, and I've decided to work some more. First of all, the homeless in Škofja Loka, if I manage to get hold of a certain women who knows all about them. But there's no hurry. I'm ready to survive without any extra fees. But if I can write a reasonable text even under the worst pressure, then everything is ok. Slowly. If I manage, I manage, and if I don't, I

DEPRA

don't. I remember once in a deep depression doing an item on an old lady who lived in a wooden cottage in the middle of the woods, more than an hour's walk from the nearest house. She lived on … I don't know what she lived on. I do know though that she was very friendly and served me schnapps. I worked very hard, but the story was pretty cool.

Renata Ažman

Tuesday, 2 August.
It began with the nightmares. In fact they were nice at first, but then they turned nasty. So I started waking up at six. I'd try to get back to sleep, but no luck.
Yesterday Andrej told me that either I don't know what depression is, or I'm a genius because even in this state I can still write. I know what depression is. And writing is usually the only thing that keeps me going. Today I'll try to get on my bike and visit the exhibition on Jakopič Avenue. In this summer heat, that's a real achievement. Better get a move on. *Project*.
The exhibition is outstanding. Aerial photographs of the Earth provide a special experience, so thanks to the Ecology Institute which prepared the exhibition. As I was riding my bike along Celovška, I watched the people. None of them seemed particularly happy, each of them absorbed in their own thoughts and problems. God knows how many of them are fighting the same illness as me.

Souls are sent to Earth to settle karma from previous lives. The purified go to heaven and begin again. All of this is God's will.
Suffering is part of life.

Many people don't believe in God, thinking that this world has rational explanations that the human mind can comprehend. But it's not like that. The human mind is wretched, while God is omnipotent.

DEPRA

Open your soul and accept everything that is meant for you.

So we really are all in God's hands and our existence in this world is ... I don't know. I'm powerless before all the great truths that the Universe reports to me. The wisdom of eternal life is the wisdom of the universe, which conceals thousands of secrets of our fates. Suffering is painful, but it's not bad. People suffering learn many truths about themselves and the world around us. So don't resist suffering, because suffering will make you stronger. You, and your soul. So they say. So suffering may even be a good thing, albeit an unpleasant one. And competing to see whose suffering is the greatest makes no sense. Everyone feels that their suffering is the worst; perhaps what one has to endure, another is spared. It seems to me that in organising our lives, we have forgotten that everything that happens, has a meaning. A meaning that may only become apparent later, much later, but it does. And the meaning of life? One day one thing, the next day something else. They say that when God closes a door, he opens a window, and new possibilities emerge. True, it's not always easy. The worst thing is if you have an innate feeling that you're pointless. And so hand on heart, I say to all mothers and fathers, for God's sake, just love your children. If you don't love them, give them up for adoption. It doesn't matter what the neighbours might say. A child is a delicate little flower in need of love above all else. Even if they eat a little less, or aren't dressed in the latest fashions, just as long as they feel accepted and loved. That was why the most important creature in my life really was that great big brown dog, which when I was sad would always lick away my tears in the middle of a lonely clearing in the dark forest, where you almost never meet anyone.

There's much you still don't know. You've got a lot to learn if you're to understand Heaven and Earth, joined in an endless cycle of life and death, the majestic system of souls and pastors, vicious world wars and peace, love and hate, suffering and joy. Earth and the universe are one, and so you are right to believe that beyond the human understanding of the world there is at least one other world, endless and beautiful, as only God's creation can be. Believe.

It's no coincidence that man has developed so much. In each generation a few geniuses are born – all of them, of course, proclaimed insane – who have dragged this world another step forwards. Many were harshly punished for their daring ideas, for blasphemy and for turning away from God. The authorities – including those in Slovenia – generally punished all those who were different. That was the way at the time of Christ, and it still is in many parts of the world. Disease, hunger, accidents, massacres and wars are just natural selection of the human race. In that respect, we're no different from other animals on Earth. God linked us into one world. Or as Darwin taught us, sooner or later

DEPRA

we will have to recognise the fact that in all probability we really have evolved from apes, but by God's will. Why do some people think that before Christ there was no God or God's will? It doesn't matter how man emerged. All that matters is that he is good and has a heart. Everything else, I leave to the creator of Heaven and Earth, who rules over us and will rule over our descendants. I've never envied anyone because they had children.
The future. What's that?
It's not so hot today, at least I can breathe.
People are miserable, sad and frightened. Many have not fulfilled their dreams. But they should just look around themselves, give a friendly smile to their neighbours and everything will get a little easier right away. Crises happen to bring people together again, opening up to each other and starting to realise how much they need each other. Man wasn't created to live alone, but should live in a pack. In a large family, ruled by reconciliation and love. But it's not like that, and time will show why God willed it so.

Go and rest. Enough words for today, let new words come tomorrow. Open your heart to this evening, and let yourself be happy. Farewell.

And it went. My inner voice. It sailed off somewhere among the clouds so that it might whisper new words to me tomorrow. I'll be waiting. Until tomorrow. Same time, same place. *Deal.*

Renata Ažman

Wednesday, 3 August.
It's pouring down outside, and it's so nice to breathe fresh air again. When it's very hot, it's hard to breathe, but today's better. I feel fairly good, and I think that this time the worst is over. I've been trapped by senseless panic for a few days, but that's part and parcel of it. Depression. It's been happening to lots of people lately. And many people have had treatment in psychiatric institutions. Even some who you'd never imagine had mental-health problems. Sadly, psychiatry is still too much of a taboo and people who've had treatment are still stigmatised. But it's nothing like that. I don't even know why I should be ashamed. If you've got mental problems, sometimes it's much worse than if you break a leg. The soul hurts differently from the body. Fear and panic are the worst, I know that much. And when – in fear – you look around yourself, the world really has no meaning.

Don't seek meaning in the outside world, because you won't find it there. Meaning lies inside you, and your heart. Look into yourself and you will find it.

The only meaning of this world is love. The love we give and the love we receive. And the more we give, the more we receive. It somehow balances out. Sometimes, when I'm depressed, I feel no love in my heart, just cold and anxiety. I recall some nice moment from the pleasant part of my story, and immediately I feel better. When the dark thoughts attack, you have to send optimistic and pleasant thoughts into battle right away. It's the only way to avoid being swept away by a tide of gloom and apathy. In fact, we all know gloom and apathy; it's just that some people handle it better and so don't need to see a doctor, while the rest of us handle these things badly and need treatment. Like physical pain, your pain threshold plays a decisive part. Some people almost feel no pain, while others are laid low by an ordinary headache. Me, I handle fear badly. I've got no weapons or countermeasures when it attacks me. What can I do?

Thursday, 4 August.
Thursday, fourth day of the week, my lucky day. ... *I felt that already this morning* ... It's still raining. The memory of yesterday still – and again – keeps me warm. I got a contract with Telekom, I'll have to pay 9000 to change subscriber. I don't understand, a simple little change in the computer, which shouldn't cost more than 1000 tolars, and they charge you the equivalent of almost four months line rental. I'm thinking that in the autumn, once everything's out of the way with the launch of Japajade, I'll rent the flat out and go travelling about. It even rhymes. On the other hand, I don't like sleeping in hostels and eating *burek*[11], if you're can find it. I like my own bed, and my bath, and kitchen, and fridge, and computer. In fact, I like being at home. As long as the phones and the Internet work, that's all I

---

[11] A savoury meat or cheese pastry snack popular in the Balkans.

need. I'd like to go somewhere where I had all of that and could still see something of the world.

Don't be afraid of challenges. Slowly but surely, continue on this path. You'll be happy.

Sunday afternoon will it seems resound with the spirit of Oliver's poems, with memories somewhere off in the distance, in the past, when night was day and day night, where he ate and drank and was happy. Memories; where would we be without them? I spent the weekend at Bohinj at Tiča's place. I got there just in time for a picnic at the doctor's. He was in a good mood, and we laughed a lot. And dinner was more than delicious. Thank you.
Monday, Tuesday, Wednesday … and so on each week, each month, each year, all of your life. Today I visited someone worse off than me, so I left him a packet of cigarettes. As I was heading back I told Sandra that I've got depression, and that grass is the only things that help me; she gave me a friendly pat and said "You've only just realised." There you go. If you've never smoked, you've got completely the wrong idea about it. It feels like you've drunk one beer, but I can't drink alcohol, so I'm half excused. Today the depression finally lifted. I won. I don't know for how long, but nevertheless, I won. That's the way. *Victory*.
It's much cooler in Ljubljana, very unusual for August. If you're going out tomorrow, better dress

DEPRA

for autumn. There goes another summer. God knows what the winter will be like.

I thought the depression would last forever. But it didn't. It's over. Unfortunately, it can always return. It's best I just accept it as part of life, *fuck it.* I needed a lot of time to get used to this unbearable feeling of fear and despair, but somehow I could never come to terms with it. I'd never imagined the world could be as black as I saw it through the eyes of a depressive. Even so, I couldn't help it. So I spent all those years living in some kind of fear of fear. I took all sorts of pills, I relied on kind words and good wishes, but the fears just wouldn't go away. Depression was usually followed by a manic phase, when I wanted to make up for everything, and it sometimes carried me off to an unknown world that I understood as long as it lasted, and then no more.

Many of the worlds our unconscious reveals to us are mysterious and incomprehensible. Don't be afraid; accept them. What people call illness is just one of the many ways to understand this, our world. Beyond the horizon is another world, and beyond that another, and another, stretching off into infinity. Accept your illness as a gift from heaven, since in truth that's what it is. Everybody must taste suffering, and it's not easy. When you're ready to accept this suffering as your own, your soul is saved. Look into yourself and answer all questions honestly. That is the way.

Renata Ažman

It's hard to accept fear, hard to accept despair, and hard to accept pain. It's particularly hard to accept your fears and mistakes. But sometimes you have to do so, if you can. A lot of the time, I've not been able to. I was afraid I wouldn't be able to work, that I wouldn't know how to pay for things in shops, that I'd have a total breakdown.

Black days come and go. So accept them as your own, since that too is life.

Rain. Still August.

It rained all night, and carried on in the morning. The cool August weather has ruined many people's holidays, but this temperature suits me much better than the usual clammy heat. It still feels like I'm wandering around a maze, looking for the exit, which I might have already found and then lost again. But I'm not the only one. At times like this, it's easy to fall into a black hole with no visible way out. Research suggests that by 2012, depression will be by far the biggest cause of sick leave in Slovenia. It's already in the top three. People are tired. We've lived through the changes in the system, and we've adapted to the new capitalism, but in the process we've lost ourselves. Fighting for work, struggling for a modest income, and hungry kids at home. How can a person be happy in such circumstances? Interpersonal relations have gone to the

DEPRA

dogs, everybody's looking out only for themselves, every day struggling to survive.
People live in communication; it determines and preserves our lives. I don't know how young people ten years from now will solve their crises, but it won't be easy. Every generation is marked by some collective trauma that it must solve in its own way. The law of natural selection applies to people too. The illness of the modern age fatefully marking our lives in this space is most likely depression. I've often asked myself where this unbearable feeling comes from, and what causes it. But I've never found an intelligent answer. But then I talked to my psychologist, and she explained that this is anger at something with which we mustn't be angry, turned inwards, against ourselves. So that's it. When I was depressed, I lost confidence in myself and in my work, and it seemed like I knew nothing and could do nothing. In depression you completely devalue everything good you've done, leading to feelings of guilt, self-contempt and terrible material collapse. I don't know how to resist it. I try everything I can think of that might help. I was talking recently to some woman who told me that she'd been depressed for eight years, and that she drank four beers every day. That was how she eased the anxiety that washed over her.

We all have our crosses to bear, and nobody can help you. Everyone's alone before God.

Renata Ažman

Still raining. The raindrops will wash off the last of the dust from the road, and in the morning the cars will probably reflect the sunlight. The little sparrows have found shelter under the eaves, but as for the people, I don't know.

When you hit rock bottom, know this: the only way is up. Don't turn back; leave the past behind. Take with you only pleasant memories and the gifts that life has given you. That is peace.

In the silence of the black horizon maybe you too will want to die. Life in depression loses all meaning, and the only thing left to you is some blind faith that the sun will shine after the rain. Have faith, and believe that depression is only a transitional phase, a life episode, from which we must learn. What depression teaches us, everybody knows. Everybody has their own story, their traumas and their suffering, so the routes out of depression are also different. Peace and quiet help some, reading the Russian classics helps others, and sport and recreation still others. When you've found your way, the pain will be easier to handle. Actually, depression is not so much pain as system collapse, a tunnel without end, a bottomless pit. The thing that helps most is if you've got someone to talk to, if you feel you're not all alone in the world. But you have to realise that nobody else can help you on the path out of depression. It is you who must slay the dragon, you alone who must find the way to live a normal life again.

DEPRA

People fear depression, in themselves or in others, so they don't accept the burden of another's misfortune. Talking to a professional, good antidepressants, therapy and faith that the depression will pass, they all also help. The deep pit of despair and pain is a terrible experience that has to be respected, and you have to be aware that it's an illness that can affect anyone.

The world is good and bad, black and white, and a whole range of shades in between. Nothing in the world is only good, or only bad. Therefore even the toughest experiences bring with them some understanding that will help you to live. Accept it, it's yours.

Bogeyman. Still August.
People are afraid of mental patients; they think we'll strangle them or something. The fear stems from ignorance and the primordial fear of the different. But recently there is no "different" in the world; we're all different. It's hard to say what's normal and what isn't any more. As the number of people with mental illness, such as depression, grows, so attitudes are slowly changing. Anyone that experiences this illness will look differently at other people with it. Many people are ashamed because they've seen a psychiatrist, as if it's something to be ashamed of. But it's not. For a long time I didn't accept the solutions offered by psychiatry. I thought I would beat the illness without any pills or psychotherapy. But it didn't happen. I had to recognise that the pills basically helped. I don't know, maybe one

Renata Ažman

day I'll be able to live without them. For now, let's just say it's not a good idea to delay seeing a doctor for too long. In the end, every day is precious and if we can get through it with less suffering, that can only be a good thing. Where does depression come from? Certainly there's an innate predisposition to this illness, but whether we actually become ill or not depends on stress and mental state. When you're at the bottom, all those negative patterns come to light, you have the worst opinions of yourself, and it seems that you can't do anything properly. Usually people whose parents created a negative self-image have problems. By definition, in childhood we believe our parents. And if we believe them, believe that we're bad, then it will be years before we can break the pattern, if we have enough support and strength.

The greatest thing we can give to children is faith. Faith in themselves and faith in God.

Even as a child I often thought about killing myself. The idea sometimes even seemed a redeeming one. But I never actually managed to kill myself. One time I tried electricity, another time, a rope. But it didn't work. Probably I was fated to live, or maybe I wasn't brave enough. Now, if I think about everything I've been through and the feelings that used to overwhelm me, I have to congratulate myself. Sometimes of course, I'm still sorry I didn't succeed. Depends on my mood. Right now, for example, I'm glad to be alive.

DEPRA

As for tomorrow, well I don't know.

Who knows? Probably best not to ask. God's plan is perfect, don't complain.

Once again I'm at the mercy – or lack of it – of the fears, which this morning sneaked back into my soul. I can't get rid of them; I don't have the strength. Please God, rescue me from this earthly life, take my soul and plant it on one of the clouds I see every day through my window. All I want is heavenly peace and a quiet rest. This morning I took a couple of antidepressants, maybe they'll help. The doctor told me to take the pills as required, and so I did. The abyss of despair waits ominously for me to return. I know it well, so I'm even more afraid. When it's like this, you don't believe you're ok. You're always looking for a rational explanation for why people want to be with you. Then comes the pleasant realisation that people are with you because they like you. Because of who you are, the energy you give off and other unclear, unspoken reasons. Then you open yourself up to love and, if you let it, there's soon beautiful, peaceful and friendly energy flowing through your energy channels. But first you have to believe. In whatever helps. But most of all you have to fight. The dragon can be beaten. At least I hope it can, because it's my last hope. Yalla!

You take life too seriously. Relax: life is a game! Play, there's no reason for you to hide in the corner and peek

Renata Ažman

out terrified from beneath a blanket. Relax. Everything will be all right. You're all right. Deal with it!

I think this is one of the keys to solving the problem, and one of the ways out of depression. Treat life as a game, believe that nothing in it is serious. And there's nothing fatal, fears are just excessive. The only problem is we can faithfully repeat it to ourselves a million times, nothing helps until we become aware of our inner essence, our child, our inner voice. That's the most important thing. Then we can let go of the rotten branch of the past that we cling to and go with the flow. That takes a lot of courage. Basically, life is about feeling good. I honestly can't see any other meaning. Maybe what children have is different. They see meaning in raising their children. On the one hand it's good, probably even redeeming. But then, when a person breaks down, it's all the more difficult. They say that wisdom comes with age, and that it's easier when you don't expect so much from life. I don't know. I'll let you know when I get there.

DEPRA

III.
<u>Healer.</u>

Today Mister Pedersen connected me to God. Mr John Kare Pedersen is a remote healer from Enebakk near Oslo. His energy helped me to overcome the fears in my head and in my chest. I felt him fill me with love, and when God laid down a little piece of himself inside me, I was forever linked to him. The only thing I ask is that he never takes this peace away. The unbearable fear has gone. For good, I hope. Three hours later, Mr Pedersen diagnosed a broken heart. Mr Pedersen is Henning's father, Henning who came to visit me in Ljubljana after a seven-year Internet acquaintance. Cool. When Henning saw me, so poor and frightened, he immediately phoned his father.
"You have to do something!" he told him. *You have to help her!*
We then held a session and I breathed, and in my breastbone I felt a splinter of glass and it hurt more and more and then ... relief. The fear left. Forever? I later phoned Mr Pedersen and asked him what had happened. "Broken heart," he said, "it's to do with your mum." Yes, I know. Henning, my friend and his son. Seven years we've been emailing each other, and now he's come to visit. Perfect timing, in the midst of a deep depression. I didn't know his father is a healer. "Manic depression is my speciality," he told me, when I called. And we held a remote session, and my fears left.

Renata Ažman

"Call me whenever you want," said Mr Pedersen.
Thanks.

Chap.
The story with Henning began one cold December night, when I couldn't sleep. At the time we were just learning to surf the Internet and to recognise the new dimensions of the new media. I was bored so I went to a chat channel. My Internet name was Nena. That's where we met. A sixteen-year-old boy with the Internet name Chap. He only confided in me that his real name was Henning a few days later. At first we chatted in a public chatroom, but we soon switched to a private channel. And so we met almost every day, describing traumas and solving problems. At the time his worst problems were maths, which he just couldn't get, and his father's anger because of the high telephone bills. All sorts of things I had to deal with were going through my head. We even celebrated New Year together once. Him on his computer in far-off Norway, me in Ljubljana. So our acquaintance developed into a friendship, and although we never met or spoke on the telephone, we trusted each other absolutely, and really liked each other. And when I saw him four days ago on platform six of Ljubljana Railway Station, I recognised him immediately. Chap, my dear friend Chap. He came at just the right time. And his father's a healer and I'm not afraid any more. Perfect.

DEPRA

"Your heart is repaired now. God believes in you," Dr Pedersen said. And: "When you've felt this peace in your heart, you don't need anything else."

My heart was pounding as Henning went to the Customs desk at Brnik airport. A boy, so talented and hardworking. He's like a son to me. He flew from Ljubljana to London, and then home to Oslo. He just slept for two days, today he was back online, but we didn't get in touch. Our meeting was a very intense experience for both of us, and now is the time to rest and reflect.

Sunday.
I was round at Jure and Alenka's, and I got a lot of stuff as well as breakfast. I always get something, a snack and something for home. Then I slept all afternoon. It's Sunday.

> Chap writes to me that his dad asked if I could write a report on the treatment and healing. I will.

Monday.
I'm going to the editorial office. And to say hello to the girls. I drank a couple of coffees, got some paper and pencils and sellotape and slips, and now my bureaucratic soul can relax for another month. I'm addicted to paper, notebooks, pads and such things.

Renata Ažman

I spent a very pleasant couple of hours at the publishers coordinating and settling the final arrangements for the press conference.

There isn't a word for what I'm feeling in my heart. Peace. Of God.

I've got a press conference for the book launch in a month; before then, I have a feeling a lot's going to happen. I hope that Mr Pedersen will come to Slovenia, hopefully with Henning as well. This month I also have to write a prearranged interview, and prepare a programme for the journalism seminar. And there's bound to be something else. *Yes.* Chap sent me a very sweet text. That cheered me up a lot. Big phone bill this month. But I can't help it. I simply *have* to communicate. This evening I forgot to go offline again, so I that the meter was running all night. I'll manage somehow. Chap, who knows that I'm trying to save money any and every way, sent me a surprised message:
"Still online?"
Yes, baby. Completely forgot. Nobody's perfect. Everything is in God's hands.

Like you and me, like us all, all day and all night, daybreak and nightfall. In my thoughts you, and you again, and that's enough for a person to ... live.

DEPRA

Or go mad. One or the other. But out on the horizon, where dreams and reality intertwine, there's no room for lies, deception or games. When it's serious, God is there; that's important. It's the only important thing. Everything else ... comes and goes ... like people ... like money ... like everything in this world. But if you believe, if you really believe, it's different: then nothing else matters and if I think carefully, it's actually the only way a person can dig themselves out of depression. Believe it.

Tuesday.
"Good morning."
Waking up this morning, I'm again listening to the cassette I already know by heart.
Chap was online last night, but we didn't chat because he was busy. Andrej promised to help me organise Mr Pedersen's visit to Slovenia. We'll work it all out somehow. Many people in Slovenia could use his help. Melita promised that I could do an interview with him for Jana[12], which is a really big deal. If people know what's happening, they'll come. Chap will make a documentary film, and we'll be doing good again. Oh God, let us succeed. If we help just one person, we've done so. The only thing I'm afraid of is that someone will turn up questioning it all, because this type of healing is not exactly common over here. The book's going to be a while yet, because I'm writing very slowly. Just a few lines a day. And even then the next

---

[12] A popular Slovenian women's magazine.

Renata Ažman

day I shorten it, change it, delete it, so it goes very, very slowly. But it's ok. A friend of mine who knows about these things says I'm writing too quickly. I think everything will be ok. Now I'm going for some meat and then a coffee at BTC. I might buy a cloth in Sarika, that really would be great. *Sababa*. Went to Sarika, bought a cloth. Was round at Alenka's for coffee. And convinced myself again that I'm not all alone in the world. It's a good feeling. I called Mr Pedersen once again, because I was afraid again yesterday. He said he'd been expecting my call and we agreed on a session at one. I have to call him once again and then everything will be ok. I think three sessions will be enough. "Healing is painful," said Mr Pedersen, "but that's the way it is." Let it be so.
... because I love you, like none before ...
My throat hurts. Mr Pedersen's ill too. Cold and flu.

... yes I feel you, because I love you ... I still protect you because I love you, like no-one before ...

It's twenty to one, another twenty minutes until the remote session. I'm feeling a little impatient. It'll pass. I lit some incense, and at one I'll light the candle from Medjugorje. I called Mr Pedersen. The session lasted three-quarters of an hour and I feel liberated from some old fears and other emotional baggage that had been building up inside me since early childhood. Fear, the need for security, the unfulfilled wish to be loved and accepted. And that was that. The fear has gone for now.

DEPRA

Mr Pedersen said it could return. If it does, I should call him right away, he insisted. And then we talked about his visit to Slovenia. He'd like to come around the third and stay until the seventh or eighth. We'll see. *Cool.* I've got to go out in half an hour, to the psychologist. I'll tell her what I'm writing now and what's going on. Just like always. I talked with the psychologist for a little over half an hour, and she told me I'm probably back in depression, because I look tired. Maybe I am. Mr Pedersen said that my state could even deteriorate during treatment, but that I was not to worry, as it's only part of the process. "Healing is a process," he often repeated to me. And as such, it takes time.

Thursday.
I'm scared again today. I had another session with Mr Pedersen at half four, and now I feel better. He told me that I still have many fears from childhood buried deep in my subconscious. And he promised me that we'd drag them out into the open, one at a time. *Thanks.*

Friday.
Scared again. For forty-five minutes Mr Pedersen sent me energy, and the fears disappeared. When I'm scared again, I'll call him. He said he has a very good feeling about me. So it's not all lost. *Sababa.*

There are many wonderful people in my life. Thank you for them, almighty God.

Renata Ažman

God is in me, God is in you. *God is all around us.*

A new, difficult day. I'm not complaining, I'm just wondering where this is heading. My view reaches to the concrete beams of the neighbouring building, with the tops of distant pines jutting up from behind them. The traffic is so loud I sometimes feel like my desk is in the middle of Celovška[13]. But the vibrations are good. Definitely. I feel good in this racket. Then I turn the radio up. I'm listening to Luky[14]. I bought it because of the design, but the music's a real find too. So another day passes and I can't remember if I've been out or not. Wait, of course I was. I went for cigarette papers, tobacco and milk. And then again to the bakery.

... And then the little white angels came to change the weather and realise one wild dream for one wild child. They wound the magic watch, and the gloomy weather was gone. Until tomorrow. Bye.

Tomorrow.

Today was tomorrow yesterday, and tomorrow will be today tomorrow.

And there we are. It's a foul day out. Holy war on the radio. Why? Where is this world going? Yet another

---

[13] One of the busiest roads in Ljubljana.
[14] A Croatian popular singer

civilisation will vanish. It will be swept away like some dog shit into the sewers of history. Why should we be any different? The world has ended many times, and I think we're very close to another end. People are confused, no money, floods, earthquakes, famine, winter. Is that not the end of the world?
So what? So nothing. We should fight for a fairer world, a world without war and injustice, a world of compassion and friendship among nations. I can already hear the song resounding from a thousand throats ... *Age of Aquarius ... I'd like all people to be happy*. But it's not like that. *The world exists, civilisations change. Ours today, yours tomorrow*. And I really don't know why we have to dramatise everything and create constant chaos. Do we really have to be confused by everything in order to understand the meaning and importance of this world? It will be our catharsis. Depression. Aids. And others. Stab in the back and the like.

Sunday, September 11, Two thousand and five.
"Good morning. And fine day."
An idea: set up a society for people with depression in one form or another. It would help with advice and in other ways. We could involve doctors, psychiatrists, psychologists, bioenergists, basically anyone who can help. I think such a society would have a lot of work. I've realised I need a break. I'd go somewhere for a rest, somewhere ... just somewhere. Or maybe I'll just rest at home: that's probably the most sensible, and certainly

the cheapest option. I've just worked out that one way or another in ten months I've written more than 450 typed pages of texts. Plenty. *Sababa*. Mr Pedersen wrote to me today. Unfortunately, he can't come to Slovenia as his wife is ill and had to go into hospital. Some other time. Truth be told, I was already a little worried about to how to organise everything in such a short time. If we had a society, we could. And this morning I found out someone has stolen my bicycle. Hello!?
It was locked, and in the bike shed.
"Good morning."
I called Mr Pedersen again. I feel like I need another treatment. We agreed on eight in the evening for forty-five minutes. All I have to do is relax at eight o'clock and open my soul to his energy.
Then I slept.
Friday morning is cold. Autumn comes slowly but surely to Slovenia. And then winter. And the year will be over. I'm thinking about God again.

... and the rain starts again, like it rains on the islands in October ...

I can't go on. It's still raining outside. The large drops are rattling off the old green shutters. The pigeons are gone, probably found some dry shelter. I'm back in the claws of the dragon. Sometimes I really wish I had some other illness.

DEPRA

Jasna saved Sunday afternoon by coming round. We talked about all sorts of things. Everything. She left in a better mood than she arrived in, and that's important. In Louise Hay's book The Power is Within You I read: *depression is anger turned inwards*. I believe it. Not it makes sense. Now many things make sense. Now many things are clear to me. Mr Pedersen promised to treat me for free as long as it takes to banish all the demons from my past causing terror in my soul. I hope so. I really hope so.

Today I found out you're not getting my texts. Shit.

And maybe tomorrow the sun will shine on this land, full of pain and fear. May the gods have mercy on us, and grant our request.
Amen.
The depression came back again, and again, and again, and so on. In a vicious circle of despair and memory, in the endless embrace of God's face here and now. I hope the angels will be merciful with me. Everybody has many lives. And my last life ended yesterday. But today is a new day. And tomorrow too. *Believe.*

Winter 2005.
The winter was hard and cold, and there was a lot of snow. Every day was pretty much like the next. And every evening I prayed that the morning would be different. And then, very slowly, that morning came.
Spring.

Renata Ažman

A late spring. But a number of difficult steps and unfamiliar paths still awaited me first.

DEPRA

March 2006.
"He knows about you and he loves you very much. He said not to worry. You are safe," Mr Pedersen told me today about noon. *God knows about you and loves you very much*, he said. *Don't worry. You're safe. Saved.* Maybe he said saved. I didn't hear him clearly. But either is good. Safe or saved. Sure. Saved from this hell? My psychiatrist says that I have to get used to my illness. Last time she lectured me, but then I asked her if it would help her if I wrote down my memories. I told her I was concerned because she was retiring. She told me not to worry. And I won't. After what Mr Pedersen told me today, definitely not. *Thank you, my angels.* Sometimes things are really bad. Sometimes I simply can't take it any more. Then I usually have to seek professional or divine help, and take a pill every few hours. The one that relaxes me. Xanax. When you reach the inevitable conclusion that you're the most lonely person in the world, Xanax stops helping. Everything becomes obvious. Should I go to Polje? If they put me in the upstairs ward, where I was last time. Maybe then. In the morning. *Or maybe I'll wait another day or so.*

Last day of March.
Yesterday was an extremely informative day. The last day of March. It started badly, so I sent Mr Pedersen a message in the morning, telling him I was lost again, and asking for his help. He wrote back that we could have a session at eleven. During the sessions, I lie on

my bed and relax. Then he heals me. He sends me divine energy. Yesterday for the first time in that way I felt loved. Unconditional love. Safe. And then I called Mr Pedersen and he told me what had happened during the healing. Archangel Michael helped him. It's very simple. "You are saved," Mr Pedersen said God had told him. I believe him. I'd be crazy not to. I don't want to spend the rest of my life paranoid. I'd rather be at peace. Some people have tried very hard for me to lose my confidence. Maybe I'll get my dreams back too? I'm not going to Polje; so today I borrowed a bike. On a bike, the world seems completely different. You can wear torn trousers and nobody notices. Actually all my trousers are torn, and if someone doesn't like it, there's nothing I can do about it. When I get some money, I'll buy a new tracksuit. For now I'll just wear the torn one, which Tiča told me is very trendy these days. The latest fashion. Torn. It'll be worse when they're no longer in fashion. Hopefully by then I'll have earned something. And then I can buy a new tracksuit.

Don't worry. You are safe. Saved.

You've got to fight through it kid!
I'm reading Jason Pegler's book A Can of Madness, and I'm right into it. Jason describes how unbearable it was in the mental hospital, and how he was then comforted. Most of all by his granny. She told him: "You poor little boy. I've felt like that, you know. Just like that. And it's a terrible thing. But I don't feel like that

DEPRA

anymore. You've gotta fight through it kid." When I got out of the mental hospital, one minute I was in safe hands, the next minute I was alone. I had nobody. The most comfort I got was ... oh, it doesn't matter. I didn't have a family. Never. Still don't. I don't belong anywhere. And I really never have. I have people I'm close to that I talk to on the phone. Basically, though, I don't go out unless I have to. And that's it. Oh, and the Internet.

The book has superb descriptions of life in a mental hospital. Jason's basically right. You soon get tired of those scenes. The one I remember best is the closed ward three years ago, when they brought me from Croatia. I was 200% manic; I imagined we were making a film and then I got a 'message' and I hit a Skoda Octavia driving in the opposite direction. It seemed like we were all one big chosen family doing good works. And if I hit the car in front of me, I'd be doing good work. I obeyed. I turned the steering wheel and boom. Now I have to pay compensation to Triglav Insurance – my insurance is not being recognised because they say I fled the scene of the accident. Six hundred thousand by November. So it goes with this illness. Maybe I ended up in Polje so that someone would deal with me? But they wouldn't. I remember what it's like. You're shut in the ward, you can't go anywhere, you can't go to bed because the rooms are locked. All that's left to do is wander the corridor and the smoking room, if you've got any cigarettes to smoke. And of course the big day room, with a table and plenty of chairs. There are magazines on the table, some with crosswords. So you can solve a crossword and think about why you're inside. In my career of three hospitalisations, I've only twice encountered genuine human contact with staff. The first time was in Split, when I chatted to a cleaning lady; the second was in Polje when I talked to the ward nurse. In fact, I don't know what took me there. Probably just another manic phase. A short one, fortunately. Now comes the depression. Fact. I'm already totally apathetic. I don't know where it's leading me, but I'm relying on the words of Mr Pedersen: "You are saved." I really hope so. Or maybe safe. Saved or safe, I don't know. I wrote another letter today. To a former friend. I doubt she'll write back, but I had to write. And I included my address. Still don't know if I'm going to post it or not.

God, you are all I have. Don't leave me, please. Please. Not you too.

Accept!
Mr Pedersen said that God loves me unconditionally, no matter what I do. Unconditionally.
"He loves you no matter what you do."
This world's not the way I remember it. Everyone's alone. If you want to survive, you have to ... I don't know what you have to do. I don't know. I've lost all criteria and I'm living from day to day. I'll take it as it comes, as long as it's pleasant and I can relax. Can't be

DEPRA

any other way. Francis of Assisi once said: accept the things you cannot change. Why should things change all the time? I'm ok and I feel good. You really don't need much to survive. And Tanja just told me that she goes to a free food store. She doesn't have anything to eat, and neither does anybody else there, so you don't feel so uncomfortable. And it's free. It's best to get there around eleven. They give food to anybody. I don't need much. Coffee and cigs and a snack. Hopefully I'll always be able to earn that with my work. I just have to get rid of this depression, which is pressing me to the ground and not letting me breathe. From time to time, but always less. Truth be told, I don't want to think any further back than yesterday. Because. God said I'm safe. *I believe him.* I also believe Mr Pedersen. I have done for some time. At times in my life, I've also believed the wrong people, and suffered greatly as a consequence. But that's in the past. My past goes no further back than yesterday morning, when I opened the window and the day rushed into me. I thought it was going to be another tough day, one for bed. Sometimes I think my life is sad. Then I realise that I've never sought stable goods and values, I've always been interested in something else. Stanka tells me that the portrait is in today's Jana. Looks like the editor likes my portraits, otherwise she wouldn't have published them. Seems I've still got it. And I won't waste any time wondering how long much longer I'll still have it – that way of thinking leads nowhere. It's completely unproductive. Thinking about the future at times like this? I can't. I want to enjoy myself. I've had enough of clarification and speculation, therapy and treatment. I'll stick to my psychiatrist's instructions: "Take your pills regularly, write as much as you can and think positive thoughts. And go for walks." It's true. I can't constantly compare myself with others. I'm not like other people. And I don't have to be ashamed of my image. If people don't like me, God help them. What do you want? If I worry about it, they won't like me any more. Probably like me even less. Vicious circle. Catch 22. Today it's also become abundantly clear that I really have to accept the fact that I'm not well. And I need to stop expecting the impossible. Because the impossible is, well, impossible. I have to keep going. I have to fight. That's all I know. Because I want to survive. And it's becoming increasingly clear that I'll have to survive on my own.

I'll do it!

I have heart, I have courage, and if I fight against the voices inside me, I'll also be fighting against those outside me. It's hard, being mentally ill. If you've never experienced it, you can't understand it. But the greater the struggle, the sweeter the final victory. At least I hope I'll win. I have to. But in my story, everything will in any case be a victory. Each day is a new victory, each morning a new attack. Or as Tanja put it to me earlier today when she was round on a visit: "Then in the morning you open your eyes, saying to yourself: Oh God, yet another day." That's exactly how I feel when

DEPRA

I'm depressed. It's happened a lot this year. But the strength is in me. Unknown strength. Everyone who knows my story tells me so. Now I'm alone, so I'm looking for someone, but in all honesty I'll probably never find anyone, because I don't believe that anyone would be ready for life with a mental patient. It's not the same as breaking your hip. It's much worse. People start to avoid you out of fear. But that's also why I'm stronger than other people – because I've been through all of that. That's where I'll draw my strength from. And I won't condemn myself any more. I am the way I am, God help me. I deserve nice and good things, like everybody in this world. Like everybody.
Fear is the devil. You can make many mistakes out of fear.
I don't know if you know what it feels like when your world falls apart and there's nothing in your head except fragments of dispersed memories, slashing and slashing and slashing into my brain and heart. I never had anyone. Just myself. And now? I'm on my own again. That's something. But I'm ill, very ill, and nothing seems to help. And when I'm depressed and those words resound in my ears, and my heart is cold, and my chest hurts, I remember the words Mr Pedersen said to me that difficult morning: "God loves you unconditionally."
Life is dragging me into some utterly incomprehensible reality, where there's nothing good any more, just bad. I haven't the will to be like other people; I'm stubbornly persisting with my collapse. And it suits me to be the

dregs of society, of a society which I hold in contempt, and I've absolutely no desire to be with anyone. I'd like to keep in touch with those who still want to keep in touch with me. As for the others ... there aren't any. Yet again, I don't give a damn about anything, and I'm now building my identity on depression. That's my reality, and I have to accept as soon as possible that there's no room in my head for sunny and gentle thoughts, only for sadness, anger and pain. How did I end up in such a state? Life. I have to recognise that this is a difficult test. Living without will or prospects. Maybe that's it though. And the idea that one day I might meet someone who'd be prepared to share that with me – today seems a hell of a long way away. Miracles can still happen, of course. But I won't change. I don't know how. Today I dreamt of war again. Second time this week.

I want to destroy myself. Wipe myself off the face of the Earth. At the same time I want to live. To suffer?

Life around me appears in strange colours. Black, mostly.

Help!
I wrote to Mr Pedersen again. "Please help me." This afternoon, I got a reply, saying that we could have a session today around half-six. During the session I felt a powerful energy flowing into my body, and then the message "Stop smoking." I didn't exactly succeed. I

DEPRA

really can't smoke cigarettes any more, so I'm rolling my own. I've got enough for one more rollup, but I'm not going to buy cigarettes. No money. I've come to the conclusion that it's all over for me. I've been looking on the Internet for a place I can live well on a pension. For free. There's nothing. Or maybe I can't be bothered looking. I don't know. I can't work. Everything just slips my mind, every idea. Everything. I don't know what'll happen to me, and I can't fight any more. I'm going to lie down. Afterwards, well, who knows? I've fucked this life up. Or maybe not. I know now why this is happening to me. I know now what I want to be and why it's dragging me back to Polje. I want to be a child with someone to care for me. As I can't see any other way to achieve this, I want to go to Polje, and I want them to look after me. Then I create great expectations and of course people become afraid. I just don't want to grow up – that's my problem – but I'll have to. I dream of the closed ward. How I lie on the floor, not wanting to get up, how they let me sleep and ... and it won't work. I just completely collapsed. But today I can allow myself this remnant of the experience of nothingness which so far in my life has shaken and scared me the most. Then I felt putting it mildly ... ah, who cares about that? Who cares about anything? I've been promised the book will be published in October. If ever. No money. People probably think I'm not trying hard enough, but they've got no idea how hard I'm trying and what's really going on inside my head. If

Renata Ažman

they knew how I struggle sometimes, they'd respect me. But most of all I should respect myself, at least a little. Today, the huge, dark-green pine tree that rises above the bypass is covered in a shroud of raindrops. It's the holidays, and I'm resting. I decided not to torment myself any more with endless accusations and questions; instead I'll live. Thank God I can lie down and watch the pine tree. It's so big I can almost see it all. It's right in the middle, through the window. Pine tree. My pine tree. It's been raining all day, and tomorrow's supposed to be wet too. It's all the same to me. All the same to everybody. I realise this can't end well, but even that's all the same to me. It's a pleasant feeling – no expectations, no promises, nothing. Absolutely nothing. Apathy.

DEPRA

IV.
Thanks, God.

Gorazd called. I met Gorazd on Skype; this morning there was a nice text waiting for me on my mobile. He lives near Maribor[15] in some place with no mobile signal, so he has to be away from home if he wants to call me. He says I should write him something. I've got no ideas, but I'll try. Something nice, he said. *I will.* I'll write to him that I'm looking for someone who would love me. And that it's nice when he calls, especially as he can't get a signal in the house and has to go far away. When he finishes work in the evening, there'll be a message waiting for him on Skype. He'll read it then. *Nice guy. I'm not afraid of Gorazd. Strange.*
Now I know why this is all happening to me. Doctor Magdič told me a while ago, and Gordana confirmed it today. Some of us have a little more to bear. God gave me a task, and I'm fulfilling it. That's the point. That's where the strength is. That's my mission: in loneliness and combat. It's the suffering that gives me the strength; the daily victory over depression that inspires me with hope that one day I'll have something other than a struggle. Or maybe the sense lies in the struggle, and there won't be any victory in the end? Every new day, every new word, every sentence is a victory. I won't give up. I mustn't. I've accepted that everything that's happening to me is my karma, and the only thing

---

[15] The second-largest town in Slovenia.

Renata Ažman

left is to fight. Not to give in to the destructive voices in my head, not to bow down before life's blows, not to humbly accept my fate, and then in the evening, when sleep sneaks into my soul, I dream those beautiful fairy-tale dreams that lead me back to some completely different world. A world of beauty and peace, a world of harmony and understanding, a world that doesn't exist, except in my dreams, and only there can I live. Today I'm going for a walk on Rožnik. With people who know what depression is. All of them.

The thoughts that even yesterday made me want me to end it all today give me strength. I'm strong. Yesterday I was still shaking like a leaf – because I thought somebody could help me. Now I know that nobody can. That I had to find the strength within myself which will lead me ... lead me where, exactly? I don't know. Nobody can know. I do know, though, that several times when I've been seriously considering suicide, one single thought would snap me out of it: "What if the fortune-teller was right?" More than twenty years ago I visited a fortune-teller. She wore black and had silver nails and long silver hair. She had an assistant, who made us coffee, and then one by one we went into the room where she read our fortunes from the coffee sediments. She said something to me that has stayed with me always. She said that I would find love in the second half of my life and that I would still be very happy. And now, when I want to kill myself, I always think of her words. What if she was right? That draws me back from the step that at the time I think would be

DEPRA

the only way to ease my suffering. Now I know that there is strength in suffering. And meaning in loneliness. Now I know I can do anything. Every step is a step forwards. In any direction, but forwards. If you want to beat depression, you have to be damn stubborn. A quick peek in the cupboard plunges me back into despair, but I'm not giving up. Clothes and shoes really are my weak point. But I can't do anything. No money. Tonight I dreamt that I was extremely rich, and everybody was dressed like in a fairy tale. Some really are like that. But my karma, it's, well, somewhere else. I have heart and courage and that's that. *The material world is not for me.* Dada told me today that she loves me. That she herself doesn't even know why, but she loves me. And I love her too. Love!
She loves me, yeah, yeah, yeah!

Gorazd called. I'm happy when he calls. I feel that we could be friends. When he said he was coming to Ljubljana and asked me to meet him at the railway station, but I chickened out. I said I wasn't sure that was a good idea. Then he said that I'm ill. That I have to break out of that habit. That I'll have to trust more. And that I should think better of him. And it's hot today in Štajerska[16]. That he's wearing short sleeves and fixing a car. If I think like that, I really will end up alone. I'm afraid of anyone who's not online. Anyone who's real, who wants to become real. Obviously I've become so

---

[16] Styria, a region in north-eastern Slovenia.

enmeshed in my inner world that I can't see out. Maybe someone will turn up who will cure me?
I wrote to Mr Pedersen that my world is falling apart, that I can't see a way out and that I'm worried. He promised to help me. Today. Hope so. I'm also writing a letter to my psychiatrist. I'm going to try to gather impressions of the events in my head over the last few days. It's been hell. And it was only Xanax that saved me from a total breakdown yesterday.

Effectin.
My psychiatrist told me that my illness has chemical roots, and so we'll fight it with chemicals. I've got new antidepressants that – I hope – save me from my torment. Effectin. I took the first one this morning, and I hope it works. It seems to me I feel better even after only one. That's basically impossible, because antidepressants only start to work after three weeks, but that's the way it feels. Maybe this really is a way out.
Gorazd.
Gorazd wants to come for a visit, but I'm not up to it. I told him so, and he was a bit hurt. The state I'm in, I'm really not ready for new acquaintances. That's just the way it is. I want to meet my other half, but on the other hand I'm frightened of every new meeting. A vicious circle. Mr Pedersen, who's treating me again, told me that two great angels helped him. I felt like I was being pricked with needles, and then slept all day. Next day I didn't feel any better. Worse, even. Mr Pedersen said that it could be a consequence of the treatment and that

DEPRA

everything would be all right in the end. He's not the only one to tell me that, so now even I'm starting to believe it. And I feel grateful in my heart. Grateful to be alive, because I am, even the way I am. That's a big step. A big step. I'm also grateful to other people in my life. And respectful. I'm even starting to respect myself. That's a big deal.
A lot for one day. It's still a full moon and today's the thirteenth. What a coincidence.

Life is a gift and I accept it gratefully, however it's been and is now.

Life is a gift and we all have our own. As it was laid down for us in the cradle, and as we're able to live it. Life is multi-layered. When you remove one layer, a new one appears underneath, even more difficult. So there's always work to be done. And then ... then, it's the end. Some people are given happy moments with their loved ones, others the loneliness of deaf concrete. But everything has to be gratefully accepted, because that's the only way to final peace. I said: "This is my path and I want to walk it." Then it was easier. As long as I was dissatisfied with every little trifle, I was unhappy. Now I'm at peace. This is my path and I want to walk it. I chose it myself, and it's hard. But it's mine. And if I lose my strength ... then it's the end. I'm not afraid. Not any more. Sometimes, when I look out the window and I don't see anything except the top of the old pine tree and the odd pigeon flying past, I wonder

Renata Ažman

about the meaning of life. At that point I always realise that life has meaning in itself. That we don't need anything else but to live for it to have meaning. That life is a miracle, and we have to respect everyone living it. Because they're alive. Because they're god's creatures who feel and think. I don't know what life's got in store for me. So much I planned, and very much hoped, but nothing ever came of it. Now I don't plan anything. Or hope. Or do I?

I wake up in the morning from a nightmare, which I accept after a coffee. Then I'm off for cigarettes. I deliberately never buy more than two packs, otherwise I wouldn't even have this walk to the shop. Then I smoke, have a coffee, drink some water – I've not been eating for two days – and think. About the past, and the future. In between I sometimes write something. I go online. I talk on the phone. And I take antidepressants and sedatives and stabilisers and such things. If the weather's nice, sometimes I head off on my bike somewhere. But not too far, and not for too long. Then I get back home, sit down, smoke and write. Čiča the sparrow keeps me company. She's happy at my place. She sings, dances, flaps her wings, sending feathers flying everywhere. I tidy up a little from time to time. But not too much. I like it as it is. Solitude has its advantages. I gratefully accept everything it brings me. *God believes in me.* I'm not interested in the outside world and I'm perfectly happy with what I've got. The flat, and myself.

DEPRA

I've not been able to get online for two days, so I don't know if anyone's written to me.

Write to me, Renata, my namesake. That I have to struggle, that there's light at the end of the tunnel and such things. Again I feel like I'm from another world.

And more and more it also feels like at the end of the tunnel there's just another tunnel.
But it's not too bad. I'm used to it already, but after a few tunnels, when you discover that there's no light after all, you get tired of hoping. What you have left takes over, and you go on. Because you have to, because you can't stop in the tunnel. Life is a struggle, and even if you don't want to struggle, you have to. Pressure from all sides: do this, do that. I can't, I don't have it, I don't want to, I don't know how. Enough. Leave me in peace. Have your capitalism; just leave me alone so that I can wait my final hour in peace. That's all I want. To sleep in the tunnel. Just that.

Where are the poems, where are the dreams?
When did we crazies die for them?

No more poems, no more dreams. Just goodbye.

Take something to remember, take something for farewell,
To comfort you when you're down.

Renata Ažman

All that is left for me is an empty memory,
Poems of unhappiness, traces of snowy footprints.
May God protect you, and guide you, and show you the way,
My prayers are with you everywhere.

If you're alone, you're alone for everything. You eat alone, sleep alone, shower alone and pay the bills alone. Sometimes it's better than doing it with someone who gets on your nerves. I know quite a few people who really get on each other's nerves but stay together so as not to be alone. Or because of children. Or the house. Or God knows why. I don't. There's a kind of pleasure in loneliness. When you've got nothing, you've got nothing to lose. Peace. And strength. And weakness. All at the same time. Outside, ambulance sirens are blazing and the noise from Celovška reminds me that alongside my existence there's another world, so very different, so very alive. I can't live in it, I can't understand it. I prefer peace. The silence of the afternoon trying to shine into my room, but I don't let it in.

I live in my own world, full of emptiness and peace. God loves me, whatever I do. Unconditionally. Even if I do nothing. And nothing's what I plan to do; I only went to the shop, where I met the lady with the red cheeks wearing a dirty coat. She bought bread and a litre of red wine. But I can't. So what if I don't have any? It's not the most important thing in the world. Eating and smoking. I can manage without either. The most important thing in the world is what you carry in your heart. What is worth living and dying for? In my life there have been many such things. People. I sometimes thought money was important in life, and I was very unhappy as a result. Now I see that money isn't important at all. All the same, you still need enough to pay the bills. Can't be helped.

Messiah.

Yesterday I went to Triglav insurance to try to persuade them to let me off with at least half ... I should start at the beginning. On 23 November 2002 at three in the afternoon I was driving totally manically along the main road through Grubišno Polje. I only found out it was Grubišno Polje later, when I had to sign the documents at the misdemeanours judge. Basically, I was driving my gunmetal grey Jeep Cherokee, wearing my sunglasses and with a German shepherd on the back seat. For some time already I hadn't known where I was. All I know is that at eight in the morning I hit a parked Golf, and as a result I was held at a police station for a long time. They eventually let me go, so I was driving along the road without any plan, and I ended up in Grubišno Polje. As I've already mentioned, I was totally manic, which means I was convinced that I was the Messiah, at least. In that state, the idea came to me: "Now hit a car." I ask: "Which one?" And the thought replied: "It doesn't matter, you just have to hit one." I didn't even think about it. I turned the steering

Renata Ažman

wheel and there was a bang. A white Skoda Octavia stopped in the middle of the road, as did I. I got out and looked to see what was happening. I was completely confused; nothing was clear. I asked if anyone was hurt, and when I found out that nobody was, I got back into my Jeep and drove off At first I wanted to park, then I forgot about it and I was caught a fair distance from the scene of the incident. The police stopped me at a crossroads, dragged me out of my car and drove me to the police station, and then on to the misdemeanours judge. All manner of things were running through my head: from the idea that the Croats wanted me to stay there to the belief that it was all just a show, and outside there'd be an enthusiastic crowd waiting to greet me ... mania is a bitch. Both are – depression and mania. Depression makes you feel like a piece of shit, while mania makes you think you're the Messiah. At the police station in Grubišno Polje they sat me down and made me wait in a little room with a handsome young inspector. I was convinced he was a forensic scientist trying to determine what sort of phenomenon I was, and he had just realised that I really was the Messiah and was just about to tell the others. He looked at some documents which seemed to me like star charts making abundantly clear that my arrival on Earth is a sign from God and that it can't be any other way. I considered my words prophetic. I was muddy and dirty, and although a psychiatrist had examined me, they didn't find any indications of insanity. They treated me like I was rational and normal, and I had to pay all the

DEPRA

fines. Madness doesn't help at all in such circumstances. They kept me under guard the whole time so I couldn't escape. I had a go at the forensic scientist, asking why the Croats had destroyed the bridge in Mostar[17]. I told him they should mass produce the sort of ashtray he offered me as I smoked in his room. I took off my jumper, placed it on the chair next to me and began to talk to him. To my jumper. I thought they would intimidate me if there were two of us: me and the jumper. I thought I was communicating with the dead, and it seemed I was being followed by the secret services. Then they released me and I found myself alone on a street; I didn't know where it led or how I would get to ... wherever I was going. I didn't even know where I was going. So I began wandering the back roads, thinking I was live on the radio and talking continually. I commented on the road and remembered the people waiting for me in Slovenia. I thought they were all in the studio following my travels. I was listening to music – various cassettes – all the time, and I completely understood individual songs. The streetlights told me who was all in the studio and what they were saying. In the middle of the night I drove to a petrol station. I filled the tank then had the idea that I had to leave all the evidence for the agent at the agreed spot. The scenario unfolded according to circumstances. I put a notepad I had with me, all my documents, including my passport, my glasses and

---

[17] A famous bridge in Mostar, Bosnia, destroyed by Croatian forces in 1993.

Renata Ažman

some money into a plastic bag, which I then left in the petrol station's fuse box. Then I went on a bit and opening the door to a room, a whole new scenario unfolded before my eyes. We were making a film, and now a stuntman would get behind the wheel of my Cherokee, while I would be taken home in disguise. Because the room also had a bed and a chair, I got undressed and placed my clothes on the chair for the stuntman to use. I lay down under the blanket but I was woken just a few minutes later by somebody who crashed open the door of the room and threw me out. I got dressed and headed to my car. I sat in it and continued driving. I came to a level crossing and – without thinking – I drove through the lowered barrier. There was a clattering sound and the windscreen shattered into a thousand pieces. I continued driving. I came to the next petrol station. I left the car there, forgetting the dog was inside. I walked across the road and had the feeling the hotel was ours, that it was run by my friends who were now waiting for me to come to my room and ... I looked for the room until I decided to take a break. I went to reception and paid for a room. I still had a fair bit of money on me. I also took three beers with me. I opened the first in the room and began talking to the streetlight. A German car turned up. That was a sign that German agents had come to help me. Then a car with Czech plates arrived. I felt increasingly safe. I talked all night with the streetlight, then I went to sleep. The madness continued in the morning. I completely forgot about the car and the dog. I went for

DEPRA

a walk nearby. All the way I was talking with someone and making up stories and scenarios. Every bush, every flower and stream, everything around me meant something. When I came to a big, stinking ditch, I thought I'd reached the end of the world, that the other world lay there on the other side of the ditch, and I mustn't cross it. The energies were very strong. I walked all day. Barefoot. When I got back to the hotel in the evening – apparently the Lučko motel on the motorway at Zagreb – I wanted some wine. I went to the restaurant and bought a bottle of their most expensive white wine. Because they didn't give me a corkscrew, out of spite I left it in the wastebasket. I still had another beer left. When I woke up in the morning, it came to me in a flash that I had to go to Split. I took a taxi and headed off to Split, where another odyssey began. When I got to the ferry port, I had the feeling I was being followed, so I left my bag and jacket on a bench in the ferry port, taking with me only the papers from the court in Grubišno Polje and some money. The court papers were the only documents I had after I left my passport and driving licence at the petrol station. Dressed in just a vest I went to the port and bought a ticket for the Brač ferry. I had an hour to wait, so I went to the market. Again, I had the feeling I was being followed and I had to cover my tracks. I took off my trainers and socks and left them on some staircase. I walked barefoot through the market; two policemen were coming in the opposite direction. They probably already had a note of my description, so they quickly picked me up and drove me to my car, and then on to the police station. Before that, they helped me buy some new socks and trainers at a stall. It seemed they only had bugged shoes. So I bought a pair bugged by the German secret service. I felt safer. We went to the police station. All I had with me was a plastic bag containing cigarettes and a ball for the dog, which I'd completely forgotten about in the meantime. They questioned me for a long time at the police station, then put me in a room under guard so I couldn't go anywhere. After a few hours I'd had enough of this and ran down the corridor; they leapt on to me and pinned me to the floor. Even before that they'd taken me to a psychiatric clinic, where they examined and released me. I'd been examined by two psychiatrists in three days in Croatia, and nobody had concluded there was anything wrong with me.

I was released from the police station around eleven. The crowd I'd expected was nowhere to be seen, and I was all alone on the pavement in the middle of Split when it began to rain. I still had two hundred kuna[18] in my pocket. I started looking for the flat where I thought my friends were waiting. I followed the red lights: it's a big town, and there are plenty. I was also looking for signs in the window lights of shuttered or half-shuttered windows. If somebody turned on a light, I thought that they were inviting me, that I had to go there. So I wandered around in the rain for who knows how long. In the meantime I was taken to the police again, and

---

[18] Kuna, Croatian currency.

DEPRA

immediately let go because they thought I was a vagrant. Then I called the number that had never let me down – *thanks* – and she was worried about me. She advised me to go to a hotel, and she'd come for me in the morning. I was shivering as I spent my last hundred kuna on the hotel, which I had to pay for in advance. We then got a taxi to the border, where there was an ambulance already waiting for me. I still thought that I was the Messiah. That the producers and angels were following me. I read the number plates, and every combination had some significance. They drove me to Polje. When I told them the story, I've no idea what they thought. But it doesn't matter anyway. I'm crazy. That's now obvious to everyone. *Except me.*

18 May 2006.

The pills are definitely taking hold. I hope so. Don't know. And Gorazd's coming to Ljubljana on Tuesday. He's expecting me to meet him at the station. I don't know if I'll actually go. I don't know what's going to happen on Tuesday. I don't even know what's going to happen in half an hour. I might fall down again and be crushed by depression, or maybe the wings of mania will carry me off to some new constellation. I don't know. I do know, though, that this is probably the end of the crisis and the new antidepressants are starting to work. For now. I'm writing – haven't done so for a while. It's May; outside, it's lovely and warm. I hope it rains tomorrow. Then at least I'd have an excuse not to leave the flat all day. And I'll stop worrying about housekeeping. It's not happening. I've got rice and macaroni. Enough. And tomorrow I get some horsemeat. I don't know what things would be like without it. *T-h-a-n-k-s*.

I feel the energy returning to me. The new pills are definitely working. Thank God.
"God believes in you," Mr Pedersen said. God believes in me. I'll make it. I don't know anything else, but I will make it. That's something, at least. I already have. I managed to beat depression that time at least for a while, and I'll do it again. And again. And again. I used to believe I'd succeed through writing. Now it's a major achievement if I manage to write anything. Maybe that's what succeeding through writing means. That gave me the courage, when Gorazd called – for the third time this week – to tell him everything that was on my mind. We talked for almost an hour. Then we agreed that he would come to Ljubljana on Tuesday, and that he'd get a taxi from the station. When, at the end of my lengthy monologue, I asked him whether – after everything I'd just told him – he was still coming on Tuesday, he said only: "Yes, what about you?"

Time for action. I have to tidy the flat, hang curtains and get some flowers. Most of all, I have to work out a menu for Tuesday. A man in the house! I told him he'd be the first man I've cooked lunch for in fifteen years. And not to expect too much. I told him he has to accept me as a friend. Then he said I'm strange. And I told him

DEPRA

... I told him everything. I have a big goal. Cooking lunch on Tuesday. And sort the flat out. I knew that I just needed a decent motive. And when I told my friend all of this, I realised again that I'm not alone in the world. First thing tomorrow, I'm going to the shop. Then Stanka's coming to pick me up and we're heading to her place. Then Mateja will come for me and take me for a coffee and flowers. Then I have to tidy myself up. For going out. Around here, they're already used to me wearing old tracksuits. I have to dress smarter to go into town. And I still have to practice for Tuesday. I'm going. To the wardrobe. Get organised. Now. This instant. Will Gorazd change his mind? Even if he does, so what? We'll see. And tomorrow is another day. I can hardly wait. My life has meaning again.

Thank you God, for such a day. And for new and old friends, and for lunch on Tuesday, and for the flower I'm getting. For all the flowers I get. The suffering was worth it.

Good morning. A bubble bath to start with. Then a nice towel. Today's the 19th of May. I'm just heading out for cigarettes, then meat and coffee. Stanka picks me up, takes me there and back, and then Gordana comes round, and Vlasta calls in the evening, and on Sunday maybe my little sunshines will come to me for breakfast. And they asked me to be the official photographer at Lara's birthday on Saturday. Lara's my niece. My little sunshine. My life has meaning.

Renata Ažman

Definitely. I'm off to print. That's the phase I like best. Print preview done, one click and you print what you've written. Till now. So I can prove I'm working. *Thank you God, for such gifts.* I can't sleep, so I'm going through old mail and I find one unopened, an invitation to the opening of an exhibition in Cankarjev Dom. On Tuesday. Unbelievable. Will Gorazd come with me? Today I talked to someone important. On the phone. It's happening. All of a sudden. That conversation, the exhibition, Gorazd, Adela – who came round for a visit this afternoon and will come. It helps her. Today I gave her healing stones. Depression. We have to help, otherwise there's nothing. It's happening. I have to tidy up the flat. Hang curtains, wash out the bath, clean the kitchen, tidy up the wardrobe. I'm pleased something has forced me into this. What should I cook? Roast beef, noodles, salad, pudding. Cool. Time to get to work!

I have will again. The antidepressants are working. Everything else too. Thank you, angels.

DEPRA

Postscript

Gorazd didn't come. I knew he'd change his mind. I'm still grateful. The effectin is still working, and there are more and more angels in my life. Thank you, God.

This is my path and I want to walk it.

Renata Ažman

Appendix

Depression is just an illness; an illness like any other

Asst Prof Dr Andrej Marušič, MD, BSc (Psych)
National coordinator for mental health at the World
Health Organisation

Mental disorders are changes in mental health as a result of which individuals or their surroundings find themselves in difficulty. The most common is depression or rather depressive disorders as disorders of mood and emotion with simultaneous changes in appearance, behaviour and thinking. The latter forms a whole range of signs and symptoms, from marked bodily and psychological changes all the way to changes in the individual's connection to the society around them:

1. physical:
    - daily mood swings worse in the morning),
    - disturbances to sleep (especially morning sleeplessness), appetite and sexual desire,
    - loss of motivation, will, energy and exhaustion,
    - inability to enjoy (absence or marked decline in desires or enthusiasm);
2. psychological:

- from dejection to a feeling of inner emptiness,
- feelings of guilt, low self-worth, despair and powerlessness,
- anxiety,
- lower tolerance, distinct impulsiveness and aggressiveness,
- disturbance to concentration and memory;

3. social:
- loss of interest in other people, and
- loss of effectiveness at work.

Of course, somebody with depression doesn't necessarily show all of these signs and symptoms. We talk of depressive disorders when certain key and several other signs appear; they have to last at least two weeks before we can talk of depression as a disorder and not a temporary or transitional state. People with depressive disorders feel it as a major burden, and the burden also exists for those closest to him or her.

Various susceptibilities influence the development of depression, from those that are primarily hereditary to those linked to the environment with which the individual comes into regular or occasional contact. Of course, there's no gene for depression, but certain individuals and their relatives can be more susceptible to it than other people. We must not overlook any possible life events that may be important triggers for depressive disorders, or that may be simply one of

many causes without having an independent causal link to depression. Depression is thus a consequence of a complex intertwining of hereditary and environmental factors:
1. long-term burdens
   - financial difficulties, unemployment etc,
   - physical illness,
   - illness of loved ones we care for, ...
2. difficulties in interpersonal relations
   - lack of trust in people,
   - personal conflicts, ...
3. life events
   - death, divorce, moving house
   - change of job, retirement, ...

At least one-sixth of the population will suffer from depressive disorders at least once in their lives; at any given time, one in twenty of the population is depressed. Due to a lack of knowledge of the reasons, causes and processes unfolding in the body during mental disorders, and the stigma attached, many individuals with depressive disorders continue to receive inappropriate treatment, if any. The diagnosis and treatment of depression must be improved by educating the professional public and other key people who encounter depressed people so that they can be directed toward seeking help, and by raising the awareness of people with depression and those close to them that depression is just an illness like any other. It's important that we explain this to people, and that they really believe it. It has to be emphasised that depression is not a sign of personal weakness and the existence of a "clear" cause of or reason for depression does not reduce the need for treatment.

Where can we turn for help if we fall ill with depression? Let's start where we normally get the most help if we're physically ill, but where advice is usually lacking during mental stress: with our loved ones. If they have noticed that our mood has been worse than normal for some time, it's worth confiding in them, as they are the people that know us best. The next step involves various organisations not directly involved in the area of health care but that provide an important source of information and advice in the event of depressive disorders. These include crisis telephone lines, which are being rapidly replaced by websites and Internet chatrooms, an increasingly widespread form of communication in the modern world. These can also be an important source of information to turn to if self-help and such advice is not enough and you need a health-care professional. Instead of medicine, some people prefer to seek help from other people, such as priests, counsellors and healers. It's impossible to say that this is not a sensible decision, since many people only need a chat or advice. Unfortunately, there are also many who need suitable professional help due to dangerous or serious depressive disorders, but who delay seeking treatment because they persist with other forms of help, thereby worsening the prognosis for their mental disorder.

Renata Ažman

It's best to start with your GP. If you find yourself in serious difficulties at night or during the weekend, you will of course turn for help to the service covering your GP, the duty doctor. General or family doctors can prescribe you medicines that are effective in treating depression (antidepressants, which actually help with the regeneration of "used" tissue and synapses, and not sedatives, which only delay the problem. Sedatives can only ever be a temporary, short-term solution; they are addictive and they increase the probability of suicidal behaviour), or even refer you to a psychotherapist, who will treat your mental problems through psychotherapy, that is through structured dialogue in which you must play an active part. He or she can also refer you to a specialist psychiatrist or psychologist, or a clinical psychologist, or you can go to the latter yourself. In any event, remember that depression is just an illness; an illness like any other.

www.ingramcontent.com/pod-product-compliance
Lightning Source LLC
Chambersburg PA
CBHW020910090426
42736CB00008B/561